HISTOLOGICAL TYPING OF TESTIS TUMOURS

HISTOLOGICAL TYPING
OF TESTIS TUMOURS

F. K. MOSTOFI

*Head, WHO International Reference Centre for the Histological Classification
of Male Urogenital Tract Tumours, Armed Forces Institute of Pathology,
Washington, DC, USA*

in collaboration with

L. H. SOBIN

*Pathologist, Cancer,
World Health Organization,
Geneva, Switzerland*

and pathologists in eight countries

WORLD HEALTH ORGANIZATION

GENEVA

1977

ISBN 92 4 176016 8

PRINTED IN SWITZERLAND

LIST OF PARTICIPANTS

WHO International Reference Centre for the Histological Classification of Male Urogenital Tract Tumours [1,2]

Head of Centre

DR F. K. MOSTOFI, Armed Forces Institute of Pathology, Washington, DC, USA

Participants

DR F. CABANNE, Centre Georges-François Leclerc, Dijon, France

DR K. GANINA, Institute of Oncological Problems of the USSR Academy of Sciences, Kiev, USSR

DR CHR. HEDINGER, University Pathology Institute, Cantonal Hospital, Zurich, Switzerland

DR V. McGOVERN, Fairfax Institute of Pathology, Royal Prince Alfred Hospital, Camperdown, New South Wales, Australia

DR R. C. B. PUGH, Department of Pathology, St Paul's Hospital, London, England

DR M. RAPAPORT, Pathology Division, Fernandez Hospital, Buenos Aires, Argentina

DR R. E. SCULLY, Department of Pathology, Massachusetts General Hospital, Boston, MA, USA

DR S. F. SEROV, Research Institute of Oncology of the Academy of Medical Sciences of the USSR, Leningrad, USSR

DR L. H. SOBIN, World Health Organization, Geneva, Switzerland

DR G. TEILUM, University Institute of Pathological Anatomy, Copenhagen, Denmark

DR E. D. WILLIAMS, Department of Pathology, Welsh National School of Medicine, Cardiff, Wales, United Kingdom

---

[1] This centre deals with tumours of the urinary bladder, testis, kidney, and prostate. The participants listed here have dealt only with testis tumours.

[2] Following a decision taken by the World Health Organization in 1974 in the interest of uniformity, all WHO-designated centres have been re-named WHO Collaborating Centres: thus the above centre is now known as the WHO Collaborating Centre for the Histological Classification of Male Urogenital Tract Tumours.

CONTENTS

Colour photomicrographs

———

ACKNOWLEDGEMENTS

The authors thank Dr I. Sesterhenn for her valuable contribution in the preparation of this publication. The photomicrographs reproduced in this volume were taken by Mr L. Duckett and Mr C. Edwards, Armed Forces Institute of Pathology, Washington, DC, USA.

GENERAL PREFACE TO THE SERIES

Among the prerequisites for comparative studies of cancer are international agreement on histological criteria for the classification of cancer types and a standardized nomenclature. At present, pathologists use different terms for the same pathological entity, and furthermore the same term is sometimes applied to lesions of different types. An internationally agreed classification of tumours, acceptable alike to physicians, surgeons, radiologists, pathologists and statisticians, would enable cancer workers in all parts of the world to compare their findings and would facilitate collaboration among them.

In a report published in 1952,[1] a subcommittee of the WHO Expert Committee on Health Statistics discussed the general principles that should govern the statistical classification of tumours and agreed that, to ensure the necessary flexibility and ease in coding, three separate classifications were needed according to (1) anatomical site, (2) histological type, and (3) degree of malignancy. A classification according to anatomical site is available in the International Classification of Diseases.[2]

The question of establishing a universally accepted classification by histological type has received much attention during the last 20 years and a particularly valuable Atlas of Tumor Pathology—*already numbering more than 40 volumes—is being published in the USA by the Armed Forces Institute of Pathology under the auspices of the National Research Council. An* Illustrated Tumour Nomenclature *in English, French, German, Latin, Russian, and Spanish has also been published by the International Union Against Cancer (UICC).*

In 1956 the WHO Executive Board passed a resolution [3] requesting the Director-General to explore the possibility that WHO might organize centres in various parts of the world and arrange for the collection of human tissues and their histological classification. The main purpose of such centres would be to develop histological definitions of cancer types and to facilitate the wide adoption of a uniform nomenclature. This resolution was endorsed by the Tenth World Health Assembly in May 1957 [4] and the following month a Study Group on Histological Classification of Cancer Types met in Oslo to

---

[1] *Wld Hlth Org. techn. Rep. Ser.*, 1952, No. 53, p. 45.

[2] World Health Organization (1967) *Manual of the International Statistical Classification of Diseases, Injuries, and Causes of Death*, 1965 revision, Geneva.

[3] *Off. Rec. Wld Hlth Org.*, 1956, **68**, 14 (Resolution EB17.R40).

[4] *Off. Rec. Wld Hlth Org.*, 1957, **79**, 467 (Resolution WHA10.18).

advise WHO on its implementation. The Group recommended criteria for selecting tumour sites for study and suggested a procedure for the drafting of histological classifications and testing their validity. Briefly, the procedure is as follows :

For each tumour site, a tentative histopathological typing and classification is drawn up by a group of experts, consisting of up to ten pathologists working in the field in question. An international reference centre and a number of collaborating laboratories are then designated by WHO to evaluate the proposed classification. These laboratories exchange histological preparations, accompanied by clinical information. The histological typing is then made in accordance with the proposed classification. Subsequently, one or more technical meetings are called by WHO to facilitate an exchange of opinions and the classification is amended to take account of criticisms.

In addition to preparing the publication and the photomicrographs for it, the reference centre produces up to 100 sets of microscope slides showing the major histological types for distribution to national societies of pathology.

Since 1958, WHO has established 23 centres covering tumours of the lung ; breast ; soft tissues ; oropharynx ; bone ; ovaries ; salivary glands ; thyroid ; skin ; male urogenital tract ; jaws ; female genital tract ; stomach and oesophagus ; intestines ; central nervous system ; liver, biliary tract and pancreas ; upper respiratory tract ; eye ; and endocrine glands ; as well as oral precancerous conditions ; the leukaemias and lymphomas ; comparative oncology ; and exfoliative cytology. This work has involved more than 300 pathologists from over 50 countries. A number of these centres have completed their work, and most of their classifications have already been published (see page 6).

The World Health Organization is indebted to the many pathologists who have participated and are participating in this large undertaking. The pioneer work of many other international and national organizations in the field of histological classification of tumours has greatly facilitated the task undertaken by WHO. Particular gratitude is expressed to the National Cancer Institute, USA, which, through the National Research Council and the USA National Committee for the International Council of Societies of Pathology, is providing financial support to accelerate this work. Finally, WHO wishes to record its appreciation of the valuable help it has received from the International Council of Societies of Pathology (ICSP) in proposing participants and in undertaking to distribute copies of the classifications, with corresponding sets of microscope slides, to national societies of pathology all over the world.

PREFACE TO HISTOLOGICAL TYPING
OF TESTIS TUMOURS

The WHO Centre for the Histological Classification of Male Urogenital Tract Tumours was established at the Armed Forces Institute of Pathology, Washington, DC, USA.

At a meeting in Zurich in 1971 attended by Dr Chr. Hedinger, Zurich, Dr V. McGovern, Sydney, Dr F. K. Mostofi, Washington, DC, and Dr L. H. Sobin, WHO, a tentative classification of testis tumours was drafted. This was then evaluated by the Centre and its collaborators, a list of which will be found on page 5.

The Centre prepared and distributed microscope specimens from selected cases of testis tumours to the participants for histological typing according to the tentative classification. In all, 250 cases were thus studied. The classification was reviewed at a meeting held in 1973 attended by the participants.

The photomicrographs reproduced as colour plates in this book are also available as a collection of transparencies intended especially for teaching purposes. To help pathologists who might wish to know the corresponding terms in French, Russian, and Spanish, translations of the classification into these languages are also given, immediately following the English version.

It will, of course, be appreciated that the classification reflects the present state of knowledge, and modifications are almost certain to be needed as experience accumulates. Although the present classification has been adopted by the members of the group, it necessarily represents a view from which some pathologists may wish to dissent. It is nevertheless hoped that, in the interests of international cooperation, all pathologists will try to use the classification as put forward. Criticism and suggestions for its improvement will be welcomed ; these should be sent to the World Health Organization, Geneva.

The publications in the series International Histological Classification of Tumours are not intended to serve as textbooks but rather to promote the adoption of a uniform terminology of tumours that will facilitate and improve communication among cancer workers. For this reason the literature references have intentionally been kept to a minimum and readers should refer to standard works on the subject for extensive bibliographies.

INTRODUCTION

This classification is based primarily on the presence of morphologically identifiable cell types and patterns that can be correlated with the clinical behaviour of the tumour. Controversial histogenetic terms have been avoided whenever possible. Because of the many similarities between testicular tumours and those of the ovary, an attempt has been made to follow closely the WHO histological typing of ovarian tumours. However, important differences in the incidence, age distribution, and clinical behaviour of the various homologous tumours excludes the possibility of a classification identical with that of the ovarian tumours.

Tumours of the testis often have a very diverse histological structure and it is therefore essential that orchidectomy specimens be examined carefully. Many representative blocks of tumour tissue should be prepared after extensive slicing of the specimen, and the non-neoplastic part of the testis, the rete testis, the epididymis, the lower cord and the upper cord, at the level of surgical resection, should be included in the sections. The specimen should not be discarded until the clinician and pathologist are agreed that the response of the patient to treatment is characteristic of the tumour that was diagnosed. In the event of an unfavourable response further sectioning of the testis may be necessary, as hitherto undiscovered types of neoplastic tissue may have been responsible for the unexpected clinical course.

Occasionally the pathologist is confronted with a germ cell tumour in a specimen from an extratesticular site, and in such cases the testes may reveal no evidence of tumour on clinical examination. Although metastases from cancers of most organs reproduce the appearance of the primary tumour to varying degrees, those from testicular germ cell tumours may be different or of a more aggressive type than the primary tumour. Thus, in a case of a metastatic embryonal carcinoma, the testis after surgical removal or at autopsy may prove to contain an apparently pure seminoma or a teratoma. In other instances the only finding is a scar in association with a focus of germ cell tumour or malignant germ cells within tubules. Such scars are often referred to as regressed or burned-out tumours. Cases in which no diagnosable tumour is found in the testis or the testis is not available for examination have to be categorized accordingly, i.e., primary site not microscopically confirmed.

Another situation that may be encountered is the presence of a germ cell tumour, e.g., a seminoma, in the retroperitoneum, without clinical evidence of testicular involvement. In some such cases the patient may be apparently cured without orchidectomy, but in other instances, particularly in association with retroperitoneal masses, the testis may contain an occult or regressed tumour, which may become clinically apparent several years later. For reporting purposes, cases of retroperitoneal and mediastinal tumour cannot be assumed to be examples of metastatic testicular cancer unless a tumour is demonstrated in the testis.

It must be emphasized that structurally abnormal testes such as cryptorchids, dysgenetic testes, and the testes of testicular feminization are characterized by an unusually high incidence of tumours and tumour-like conditions. In cryptorchids, foci of seminiferous tubules often form nodules that may be confused with Sertoli cell tumours. Also, cryptorchids are particularly prone to develop germ cell tumours, most commonly seminomas, even after an orchidopexy has been performed. Dysgenetic testes are often characterized by confusing microscopical patterns of germ cell arrangement, some of which are possibly precancerous; these testes are often involved by gonadoblastomas and germ cell tumours.

The age of the patient provides a clue to the most likely type of testicular tumour that may be present. The majority occur between the ages of 20 and 50 years. Before the age of puberty seminoma is extremely uncommon and yolk sac tumours and the better differentiated types of teratoma are the usual tumours. Malignant lymphoma is typically a tumour of the older patient, but may also occur in younger individuals.

Synonyms are listed only if they have been widely used or if they are considered to be important for an understanding of the disease. In such cases, the preferred term is given first, followed by the synonym in square brackets.

HISTOLOGICAL CLASSIFICATION
OF TESTIS TUMOURS

I. GERM CELL TUMOURS

A. TUMOURS OF ONE HISTOLOGICAL TYPE

1. Seminoma
2. Spermatocytic seminoma
3. Embryonal carcinoma
4. Yolk sac tumour [embryonal carcinoma, infantile type; endodermal sinus tumour]
5. Polyembryoma
6. Choriocarcinoma
7. Teratomas
   (a) Mature
   (b) Immature
   (c) With malignant transformation

B. TUMOURS OF MORE THAN ONE HISTOLOGICAL TYPE

1. Embryonal carcinoma and teratoma [teratocarcinoma]
2. Choriocarcinoma and any other types (specify type)
3. Other combinations (specify)

II. SEX CORD/STROMAL TUMOURS

A. WELL-DIFFERENTIATED FORMS

1. Leydig cell tumour
2. Sertoli cell tumour
3. Granulosa cell tumour

B. MIXED FORMS (specify)

C. INCOMPLETELY DIFFERENTIATED FORMS

— 15

III. TUMOURS AND TUMOUR-LIKE LESIONS CONTAINING BOTH GERM CELL AND SEX CORD/STROMAL ELEMENTS

A. GONADOBLASTOMA

B. OTHERS

IV. MISCELLANEOUS TUMOURS

A. CARCINOID

V. LYMPHOID AND HAEMATOPOIETIC TUMOURS

VI. SECONDARY TUMOURS

VII. TUMOURS OF COLLECTING DUCTS, RETE, EPIDIDYMIS, SPERMATIC CORD, CAPSULE, SUPPORTING STRUCTURES, AND APPENDICES

A. ADENOMATOID TUMOUR

B. MESOTHELIOMA

C. ADENOMA

D. CARCINOMA

E. MELANOTIC NEURO-ECTODERMAL TUMOUR

F. BRENNER TUMOUR

G. SOFT TISSUE TUMOURS

  1. Embryonal rhabdomyosarcoma
  2. Others

VIII. UNCLASSIFIED TUMOURS

IX. TUMOUR-LIKE LESIONS

A. EPIDERMAL [EPIDERMOID] CYST

B. NONSPECIFIC ORCHITIS

C. NONSPECIFIC GRANULOMATOUS ORCHITIS

D. SPECIFIC ORCHITIS

E. MALAKOPLAKIA

F. FIBROMATOUS PERIORCHITIS

G. SPERM GRANULOMA

H. LIPOGRANULOMA

I. ADRENAL RESTS

J. OTHERS

CLASSIFICATION HISTOLOGIQUE
DES TUMEURS DU TESTICULE

I. TUMEURS GERMINALES

A. TUMEURS À UNE SEULE COMPOSANTE HISTOLOGIQUE

1. Séminome
2. Séminome spermatocytaire
3. Carcinome embryonnaire
4. Tumeur vitelline [carcinome embryonnaire, type infantile; tumeur du sinus endodermique]
5. Polyembryome
6. Choriocarcinome
7. Tératome [dysembryome]
   (*a*) mature
   (*b*) immature
   (*c*) cancérisé

B. TUMEURS À PLUSIEURS COMPOSANTES HISTOLOGIQUES

1. Carcinome embryonnaire et tératome [tératocarcinome]
2. Choriocarcinome et tout autre type de tumeurs (le préciser)
3. Autres combinaisons (les préciser)

II. TUMEURS DES CORDONS SEXUELS ET DU STROMA GONADIQUE

A. FORMES BIEN DIFFÉRENCIÉES

1. Tumeur à cellules de Leydig
2. Tumeur à cellules de Sertoli
3. Tumeur de la granulosa

B. FORMES INTRIQUÉES (les préciser)

C. FORMES INCOMPLÈTEMENT DIFFÉRENCIÉES

III. TUMEURS ET PSEUDOTUMEURS
CONTENANT À LA FOIS DES CELLULES GERMINALES
ET DES CELLULES DES CORDONS SEXUELS ET DU
STROMA GONADIQUE: TUMEURS DE L'ÉBAUCHE GONADIQUE

A. GONADOBLASTOME

B. AUTRES TUMEURS

IV. TUMEURS VARIÉES

A. CARCINOÏDE

V. TUMEURS DES TISSUS LYMPHOÏDES
ET HÉMATOPOIÉTIQUES

VI. TUMEURS SECONDAIRES

VII. TUMEURS DES CANAUX EXCRÉTEURS, DU RÈTE,
DE L'ÉPIDIDYME, DU CORDON SPERMATIQUE, DE LA
CAPSULE, DES TISSUS DE SOUTIEN ET DES ANNEXES

A. TUMEUR ADÉNOMATOÏDE

B. MÉSOTHÉLIOME

C. ADÉNOME

D. CARCINOME

E. TUMEUR MÉLANOTIQUE NEURO-ECTODERMIQUE [PROGONOME MÉLANOTIQUE]

F. TUMEUR DE BRENNER

G. TUMEUR DES TISSUS MOUS

1. Rhabdomyosarcome embryonnaire
2. Autres tumeurs

VIII. TUMEURS NON CLASSÉES

IX. LÉSIONS PSEUDO-TUMORALES

A. KYSTE ÉPIDERMOÏDE

B. ORCHITE NON SPÉCIFIQUE

C. ORCHITE GRANULOMATEUSE NON SPÉCIFIQUE

D. ORCHITE SPÉCIFIQUE

E. MALACOPLASIE

F. PÉRIORCHITE FIBROMATEUSE

G. GRANULOME SPERMATIQUE

H. LIPOGRANULOME

I. VESTIGE SURRÉNALIEN

J. AUTRES LÉSIONS

ГИСТОЛОГИЧЕСКАЯ КЛАССИФИКАЦИЯ ОПУХОЛЕЙ ЯИЧКА

I. ГЕРМИНОГЕННЫЕ ОПУХОЛИ

A. Опухоли одного гистологического типа

1. Семинома
2. Сперматоцитарная семинома
3. Эмбриональный рак
4. Опухоль желточного мешка [эмбриональный рак инфантильного типа; опухоль эндодермального синуса]
5. Полиэмбриома
6. Хорионэпителиома
7. Тератомы
   (*a*) зрелая
   (*b*) незрелая
   (*c*) с злокачественной трансформацией

B. Опухоли более чем одного гистологического типа

1. Эмбриональный рак и тератома [тератокарцинома]
2. Хорионэпителиома и другие виды (уточнить какие)
3. Другие комбинации (уточнить какие)

II. ОПУХОЛИ СТРОМЫ ПОЛОВОГО ТЯЖА

A. Хорошо дифференцированные формы

1. Опухоли из клеток Лейдига
2. Опухоли из клеток Сертоли
3. Гранулезоклеточные опухоли

B. Смешанные формы (уточнить какие)

C. Неполностью дифференцированные формы

III. ОПУХОЛИ И ОПУХОЛЕПОДОБНЫЕ ПОРАЖЕНИЯ, СОДЕРЖАЩИЕ ГЕРМИНАТИВНЫЕ КЛЕТКИ И ЭЛЕМЕНТЫ СТРОМЫ ПОЛОВОГО ТЯЖА

A. Гонадобластома

B. Другие

IV. СМЕШАННЫЕ ОПУХОЛИ

A. Карциноид

V. ОПУХОЛИ ЛИМФОИДНОЙ И КРОВЕОБРАЗУЮЩЕЙ ТКАНЕЙ

VI. ВТОРИЧНЫЕ ОПУХОЛИ

VII. ОПУХОЛИ ПРЯМЫХ КАНАЛЬЦЕВ, СЕТИ ЯИЧКА ПРИДАТКА, СЕМЕННОГО КАНАТИКА, КАПСУЛЫ, ПОДДЕРЖИВАЮЩИХ СТРУКТУР И РУДИМЕНТАРНЫХ ОБРАЗОВАНИЙ

A. Аденоматоидная опухоль

B. Мезотелиома

C. Аденома

D. Рак

E. Меланотическая нейроэктодермальная опухоль

F. Опухоль Бреннера

G. Мягкотканные опухоли

    1. Эмбриональная рабдомиосаркома

    2. Другие

VIII. НЕКЛАССИФИЦИРУЕМЫЕ ОПУХОЛИ

IX. ОПУХОЛЕПОДОБНЫЕ ПОРАЖЕНИЯ

A. Эпидермальная [эпидермоидная] киста

B. Неспецифический орхит

C. Неспецифический грануломатозный орхит

D. Специфический орхит

E. Малакоплакия

F. Фиброматозный периорхит

G. Сперматоцитарная гранулома

H. Липогранулома

I. Надпочечниковые остатки

J. Другие

CLASIFICACION HISTOLOGICA
DE LOS TUMORES DEL TESTICULO

I. TUMORES DE CELULAS GERMINATIVAS

A. TUMORES DE UN SOLO TIPO HISTOLÓGICO

 1. Seminoma
 2. Seminoma espermatocítico
 3. Carcinoma embrionario
 4. Tumor de saco vitelino [carcinoma embrionario, tipo infantil; tumor del seno endodérmico]
 5. Poliembrioma
 6. Coriocarcinoma
 7. Teratomas
    (*a*) Maduro
    (*b*) Inmaduro
    (*c*) Con transformación maligna

B. TUMORES DE MAS DE UN TIPO HISTOLÓGICO

 1. Carcinoma embrionario y teratoma [teratocarcinoma]
 2. Coriocarcinoma y cualquier otro tipo (especificar tipo)
 3. Otras combinaciones (especificar)

II. TUMORES DE LOS CORDONES SEXUALES
Y DEL ESTROMA

A. FORMAS BIEN DIFERENCIADAS

 1. Tumor de células de Leydig
 2. Tumor de células de Sertoli
 3. Tumor de células de la granulosa

B. FORMAS MIXTAS (especificar)

C. FORMAS INCOMPLETAMENTE DIFERENCIADAS

III. TUMORES Y LESIONES SEUDOTUMORALES CONTENIENDO AMBOS CELULAS GERMINATIVAS Y ELEMENTOS DE LOS CORDONES SEXUALES Y DEL ESTROMA

A. GONADOBLASTOMA

B. OTROS

IV. TUMORES VARIOS

A. CARCINOIDE

V. TUMORES LINFOIDES Y HEMATOPOIETICOS

VI. TUMORES SECUNDARIOS

VII. TUMORES DE CONDUCTOSCOLECTORES, RETE, EPIDIDIMO, CORDON ESPERMATICO, CAPSULA, ESTRUCTURAS DE SOPORTE Y APENDICES

A. TUMOR ADENOMATOIDE

B. MESOTELIOMA

C. ADENOMA

D. CARCINOMA

E. TUMOR MELANÓTICO NEURO-ECTODÉRMICO

F. TUMOR DE BRENNER

G. TUMOR DE TEJIDOS BLANDOS

1. Rabdomiosarcoma embrionario
2. Otros

VIII. TUMORES NO CLASIFICADOS

IX. LESIONES SEUDOTUMORALES

A. QUISTE EPIDÉRMICO [EPIDERMOIDE]

B. ORQUITIS NO ESPECÍFICA

C. ORQUITIS GRANULOMATOSA NO ESPECÍFICA

D. ORQUITIS ESPECÍFICA

E. MALACOPLAQUIA

F. PERIORQUITIS FIBROMATOSA

G. GRANULOMA ESPERMÁTICO

H. LIPOGRANULOMA

I. RESTOS ADRENALES

J. OTROS

DEFINITIONS
AND EXPLANATORY NOTES

I. GERM CELL TUMOURS

The large majority of primary testicular tumours originate from germ cells and contain one or more of the following histological types: seminoma, spermatocytic seminoma, embryonal carcinoma, yolk sac tumour, teratoma, and choriocarcinoma. The classification of germ cell tumours must take into consideration the potential of neoplastic germ cells to form a wide range of cells, tissues, or organs recapitulating embryonic and extra-embryonic development.

Nearly half the germ cell tumours of the testis contain more than one tumour type and the metastases may be of different types from the primary growth.

One of the component types of tumour may be quite small and yet determine the clinical course. It is therefore necessary to take many blocks of tissue for adequate histological sampling.

Germ cell tumours are also found in the ovary, the retroperitoneum, the mediastinum, and the pineal region.

A. TUMOURS OF ONE HISTOLOGICAL TYPE

1. *Seminoma* (Fig. 1-14): A tumour of fairly uniform cells, typically with clear cytoplasm and well-defined cell borders, resembling primitive germ cells.

The cytoplasm typically contains glycogen, a feature that may be helpful in distinguishing this tumour from spermatocytic seminoma and lymphoma. A characteristic feature of seminoma is the lymphocytic infiltration of the stroma. A variable amount of fibrous tissue may be present, resulting in an alveolar pattern. Occasionally the stromal reaction consists of tuberculoid granulomas with Langhans' giant cells.

The tumour may be in the form of circumscribed masses or it may be diffusely infiltrative. Neoplastic cells may be seen within adjacent testicular tubules. Such an intratubular seminoma is occasionally observed in association with other germ cell tumours.

Tumours with many mitoses (i.e., 3 per high power field) and/or considerable nuclear variation have been designated *anaplastic* and are claimed to have a higher incidence of metastases. Attention should be drawn to such tumours by recording their degree of mitotic activity.

Tumour giant cells or syncytial masses resembling syncytiotrophoblast may be present. Although the latter may sometimes be shown to contain chorionic gonadotrophin, their presence should not be interpreted as indicating choriocarcinoma unless they are associated with cytotrophoblast.

2. *Spermatocytic seminoma* (Fig. 15-19): A distinctive tumour composed of cells that vary in size from lymphocyte-like cells to giant cells of about 100 μm in diameter. The bulk of the tumour, however, is composed of cells of intermediate size.

The cells of this tumour have eosinophilic cytoplasm and round nuclei. The nuclei of larger cells may have a filamentous or spireme pattern not unlike that seen in spermatogenesis. Mitoses are often very numerous, but metastases are seldom reported.

Other features in which this tumour differs from classical seminoma are the absence of intracellular glycogen and the absence of a lymphocytic or granulomatous stroma.

3. *Embryonal carcinoma* (Fig. 20-34): A tumour composed of cells of primitive epithelial appearance, often with clear cytoplasm, growing in a variety of patterns—acinar, tubular, papillary, and solid.

The stroma may contain primitive mesenchyme but its presence does not indicate a diagnosis of teratoma. Lymphocytic and granulomatous reactions are infrequent.

Solid embryonal carcinomas may simulate seminoma. The absence of a lymphocytic stromal infiltrate is helpful in distinguishing between the two. The cell borders in embryonal carcinoma are usually much less distinct than those in seminoma. Some areas of embryonal carcinoma may resemble cytotrophoblast.

4. *Yolk sac tumour [embryonal carcinoma, infantile type ; endodermal sinus tumour]* (Fig. 35-44): A tumour characterized by cells of primitive appearance, growing typically in a loose vacuolated network. Reticular, tubular, papillary, and solid patterns may be present.

The cells vary from columnar or cuboidal to flattened endothelial-like cells and may have a clear vacuolated cytoplasm. The tumour contains varying amounts of mucin, glycogen, and fat.

Distinctive perivascular structures resembling the endodermal sinuses of the rat placenta (Fig. 43), cysts resembling yolk sac vesicles, and both intracellular and extracellular PAS-positive hyaline globules may be present.

Elongated cells with some of the features of smooth muscle may be present in the stroma, but this should not be interpreted as representing a teratomatous element.

Yolk sac tumour is the characteristic and most common testicular tumour of infants and young children and has also been known by the following terms: embryonal carcinoma, infantile type; endodermal sinus tumour; embryonal adenocarcinoma; clear cell adenocarcinoma; orchioblastoma. Comparable tumours may occur in adults, in which case they are usually associated with other germ cell tumours.

5. *Polyembryoma* (Fig. 45-47): A tumour composed predominantly of embryoid bodies.

Embryoid bodies are structures containing a disk and cavities surrounded by loose mesenchyme simulating an embryo of about two weeks' gestation. Tubular structures (resembling endoderm) and syncytiotrophoblastic elements may be present.

Polyembryoma as defined is extremely rare. Embryoid bodies are found more often within embryonal carcinoma and teratoma.

6. *Choriocarcinoma* (Fig. 48-50): A highly malignant tumour composed of elements identical with syncytiotrophoblast and cytotrophoblast.

This category is reserved for the very rare pure forms of this tumour. When choriocarcinoma occurs in combination with other germ cell tumours it should be assigned to category I.B.2. (see page 31).

The only criterion by which cytotrophoblastic cells can be recognized is their intimate relationship with syncytiotrophoblastic cells. Syncytial cells alone are not sufficient for the diagnosis. There is no definite villus formation of placental type, i.e., with stromal cores, although villus-like structures with syncytiotrophoblast surrounding masses of cytotrophoblast are sometimes seen, particularly at the advancing edge of the tumour. Villus formation is not essential for the diagnosis.

The tumour masses are frequently related to thin-walled vascular spaces and the tumour is usually very haemorrhagic.

Serum and urinary levels of chorionic gonadotrophin are almost invariably elevated in the presence of choriocarcinoma but this can also occur with other germ cell tumours in the absence of demonstrable choriocarcinoma.

7. *Teratoma :* A tumour that is, typically, composed of several types of tissue representing different germinal layers (endoderm, mesoderm, and ectoderm).

When multiple tissues representing only one germ layer, e.g., skin and brain, are present, it is usual to regard such a tumour in the testis as a teratoma.

If a single type of differentiated tissue, e.g., cartilage, is associated with seminoma or embryonal carcinoma, that tissue should then be considered to be teratomatous. However, epidermal cysts and carcinoid tumours occurring alone should be classified separately (see below).

(*a*) *Mature teratoma* (Fig. 51-56): A teratoma composed exclusively of well-differentiated tissues, which may be arranged in an organoid manner. Mitoses are absent or very rare.

In spite of the apparent maturity of the tissues in mature teratomas, the clinical course in adults is unpredictable. The prognosis in infants and young children, however, is usually favourable.

A careful examination should always be made to exclude immature components (category I.A.7.b) or small foci of other germ cell tumours (category I.B).

Dermoid cysts (Fig. 56) similar to those of the ovary are rare in the testis. These cysts should be diagnosed as such and classified under mature teratoma. Dermoid cysts should be distinguished from epidermal cysts (Fig. 57) which are lined by squamous epithelium without skin appendages. If the latter is adjacent to a scar or a focus of a recognized type of tissue, e.g., cartilage, it should be classified as teratoma; if it occurs alone, it is classified as an epidermal cyst (see p. 36, category IX.A).

(*b*) *Immature teratoma* (Fig. 58-62): A teratoma in which there are incompletely differentiated tissues. Mitoses are typically present.

Varying amounts of mature elements are usually present in immature teratomas.

(*c*) *Teratoma with malignant transformation* (Fig. 63-64): An extremely rare form of teratoma containing a malignant component of a type typically encountered in other organs and tissues. Sarcoma, squamous cell carcinoma, and adenocarcinoma are its commonest forms.

Carcinoid in a teratoma should be classified here. The malignant component should be specified in the diagnosis, e.g. " teratoma with squamous cell carcinoma ".

B. TUMOURS OF MORE THAN ONE HISTOLOGICAL TYPE: Tumours in which more than one of the above histological types are present.

Any combination of histological types may occur. The relative amounts of each component should be estimated and recorded as far as possible in the description of the tumour, since this information may be significant.

Seminoma is frequently combined with other germ cell tumours and in such instances is sometimes confined to the tubules. The prognosis depends upon the other components. Typically, spermatocytic seminoma occurs in pure form.

From the points of view of frequency and prognosis, two combinations are most important:

1. *Embryonal carcinoma and teratoma [teratocarcinoma]* (Fig. 65-69)

   This is the most frequent combination.

2. *Choriocarcinoma and any other type of germ cell tumour* (Fig. 70-71)

   This combination has a grave prognosis.

3. *Other combinations* (Fig. 72-73)

   The components should be specified.

   Scars in association with germ cell tumours are discussed on page 13.

   Intratubular malignant germ cells (Fig. 74) may be present with other identifiable germ cell tumours or scars. If such intratubular cells are not associated with another tumour or scar, the lesion should be classified under the category they resemble most, e.g., seminoma.

II. SEX CORD/STROMAL TUMOURS

These rare tumours have also been designated androblastomas, gonadal stromal tumours, mesenchymomas, and sex cord–mesenchymal tumours. The name given to this group of tumours does not indicate a preference for any particular concept of testicular embryogenesis. Throughout this section the aim has been to have a close parallelism with the WHO terminology and classification of ovarian tumours.[1]

A small proportion of these tumours, almost always in adults, metastasize, but it may not be possible on histological grounds to forecast their behaviour. It has been suggested, however, that the presence of numerous mitoses, particularly abnormal forms, necrosis, vascular invasion, and extension to rete testis, tunica, and epididymis may be significant. There may be a dense fibrous stroma, calcification, and metaplastic bone formation.

---

[1] See: Serov, S. F., Scully, R. E. & Sobin, L. H. (1973) *Histological typing of ovarian tumours*, Geneva, World Health Organization (*International Histological Classification of Tumours*, No. 9).

A. WELL-DIFFERENTIATED FORMS

1. *Leydig cell tumour* [*interstitial cell tumour*] (Fig. 75-87): A tumour composed of Leydig cells, which corresponds to the hilus cell tumour of the ovary.

When present, Reinke's crystals are helpful in the identification of Leydig cells. Lipofuscin is often present in Leydig cells.

Leydig cell tumours have to be distinguished from the nodular aggregations of Leydig cells found in the testes of persons with Klinefelter's syndrome.

In children these tumours are associated with macrogenitosomia. In adults gynaecomastia and other signs of feminization may be present.

Tumours and tumour-like proliferations of cells resembling both Leydig and adrenocortical cells, typically bilateral, may occur in congenital adrenogenital syndrome. Clinical and biochemical data are necessary to determine whether the lesion is a manifestation of the adrenogenital syndrome.

2. *Sertoli cell tumour* (Fig. 89-94): A tumour composed of Sertoli cells arranged in well-defined tubules.

These tumours correspond to the tubular androblastoma or Sertoli cell tumour of the ovary, although the morphological similarity is not exact in many instances.

The tubules forming this tumour may have a distinct lumen or they may appear solid as in the prepubertal testis, and their cells may contain varying amounts of lipid. When the intratubular Sertoli cells are distended with lipid the tumour corresponds to the " tubular androblastoma with lipid storage " of the ovary. Sometimes the intratubular cells have eosinophilic granular cytoplasm.

Coiled tubules lined by Sertoli cells found in undescended testes (Fig. 88) are not neoplastic and should not be mistaken for a Sertoli cell tumour.

A number of adults with Sertoli cell tumours have gynaecomastia and other signs of feminization.

In the rare syndrome of testicular feminization (androgen-insensitivity syndrome) the patients have an XY genotype and are well-developed phenotypic females whose testes are usually found in the groin or abdomen. The testes may contain tumour-like masses of Sertoli cells and Leydig cells that could perhaps be more properly regarded as hamartomas. Sertoli cell lesions (" tubular adenomas ") of very large size (up to 25 cm in diameter) can also occur. About 25% of patients over the age of 30 years develop seminoma.

3. *Granulosa cell tumour* (Fig. 95)

This is morphologically similar to the ovarian counterpart. It is exceedingly rare in the testis.

B. MIXED FORMS (Fig. 96-98)

These include combinations of differentiated cell types, e.g., Sertoli and Leydig cell tumours. Their components should be specified.

C. INCOMPLETELY DIFFERENTIATED FORMS (GONADAL STROMAL TUMOURS, ANDROBLASTOMA) (Fig. 99-106)

These include intermediate and poorly differentiated tumours similar to those found in the ovary.[1]

The tumours of this group can be composed of undifferentiated tissue, in which attempts at tubule formation may be discerned. Elements resembling theca cells may constitute part or all of the tumour.

About 10% of these tumours are clinically malignant.

III. TUMOURS AND TUMOUR-LIKE LESIONS CONTAINING BOTH GERM CELL AND SEX CORD/STROMAL ELEMENTS

There is a predisposition in dysgenetic gonads and undescended testes to the development of tumours or tumour-like proliferations of both germ cell and sex cord/stromal elements.

A. GONADOBLASTOMA (Fig. 107-109): A tumour composed of two principal cell types, large germ cells similar to those of seminoma and small cells resembling immature Sertoli and granulosa cells; elements resembling Leydig cells may also be present.

Hyaline bodies that simulate Call-Exner bodies are typically present, and foci of calcification are common. In some tumours the nests composed of the two major cell types are circumscribed, but in others the germ cells transgress the margins of the nests and grow as a seminoma. Certain tumours appear in the form of a seminoma or a more highly malignant type of germ cell tumour with only small foci of gonadoblastoma within them or at their margins. The type of germ cell tumour should be specified because of therapeutic implications. The occurrence of two distinct tumours, e.g., Leydig cell tumour and seminoma, should not be considered as a gonadoblastoma.

Gonadoblastomas arise almost exclusively in patients with dysgenetic gonads, most of whom are phenotypic females and almost all of whom are chromatin-negative and have a Y-chromosome.

---

[1] See: Serov, S. F., Scully, R. E. & Sobin, L. H. (1973) *Histological typing of ovarian tumours*, Geneva, World Health Organization (*International Histological Classification of Tumours*, No. 9).

Cases without known chromosomal abnormalities have been seen. These have a more diffuse growth pattern than the typical gonadoblastoma. Hyaline bodies are inconspicuous or absent. These tumours have been referred to as " atypical gonadoblastomas " (Fig. 109).

B. OTHERS

In some instances structures may occur resembling primitive gonads without distinct tumour formation. These have been regarded as hamartomas.

IV. MISCELLANEOUS TUMOURS

A. CARCINOID (Fig. 110)

This may be a component of a teratoma and should then be classified in category I.A.7. and appropriately designated; however, it may occur in pure form either in a primary growth (classified in category IV.A.) or as a metastasis (classified in category VI). The distinction between the last two may be difficult.

V. LYMPHOID AND HAEMATOPOIETIC TUMOURS (Fig. 111-114)

Testicular enlargement may be the initial manifestation of lymphomas or plasmacytoma. This category is reserved for such tumours.

Characteristic features of testicular lymphomas are extensive intertubular infiltration, bilaterality, and paratesticular involvement. Reticulosarcoma is sometimes mistaken for seminoma or embryonal carcinoma. The nuclear/cytoplasmic ratio is greater in reticulosarcoma than in seminoma or embryonal carcinoma.

VI. SECONDARY TUMOURS (Fig. 115-116)

Rarely, testicular enlargement due to metastatic tumour is the first indication of extragonadal cancer. Any tumour that does not have the typical appearance of a testicular tumour should be suspected of being a secondary tumour.

VII. TUMOURS OF COLLECTING DUCTS, RETE, EPIDIDYMIS, SPERMATIC CORD, CAPSULE, SUPPORTING STRUCTURES, AND APPENDICES

A variety of uncommon tumours is found in these sites. The topography of the tumour is important in determining its nature, and multiple sections may be necessary. This is particularly the case in lesions of the appendices.

A. ADENOMATOID TUMOUR (Fig. 117-119): A benign tumour in which there are numerous spaces and clefts lined or traversed by cells that may resemble endothelium, epithelium, or mesothelium. The fibrous stroma is often hyalinized and there may be lymphocytic infiltrates. Smooth muscle is often present but should not be taken as evidence of invasion. The tumour is seen in the epididymis more frequently than in the capsule and spermatic cord.

B. MESOTHELIOMA (Fig. 121-123)

Apart from adenomatoid tumour, which is regarded as mesothelial, neoplastic proliferations of mesothelium occur that may be benign or malignant, but sometimes the distinction between these two may be difficult.

Hyperplasias, often papillary, and sequestrations of mesothelium in inflammatory lesions must not be mistaken for neoplasms (Fig. 120).

C. ADENOMA (Fig. 124-126): A benign epithelial tumour forming glandular or papillary structures.

Adenomas occur in the collecting ducts, rete and epididymis. Those in the epididymis are usually composed of glycogen-rich clear cells.

Amongst the tumours of this type are those that occur in the von Hippel-Lindau complex.

Adenomas should not be mistaken for metastatic carcinoma.

D. CARCINOMA (Fig. 127-130): A malignant epithelial tumour forming glandular or papillary structures.

Carcinomas occur in the collecting ducts, rete and epididymis.

Because of their extreme rarity, these tumours can be diagnosed only when the possibility that the tumour is not a secondary has been excluded.

E. MELANOTIC NEURO-ECTODERMAL TUMOUR (Fig. 131-132): A tumour arising in the epididymis and occasionally in the testis. The tumour consists of varying proportions of two cell types—epithelium-like cells, often arranged in strands, and small, darkly staining lymphocyte-like cells—in a cellular fibrous stroma. Melanin is found within the epithelium-like cells, and to a lesser extent within the lymphocyte-like cells.

This tumour is also known as retinal anlage tumour, melanotic hamartoma, and melanotic progonoma.

F. BRENNER TUMOUR

This tumour is identical with its ovarian counterpart but is exceedingly rare in the testis.

G. Soft tissue tumours

Soft tissue tumours are classified according to the scheme devised by the International Reference Centre for the Histological Classification of Soft Tissue Tumours.[1]

1. *Embryonal rhabdomyosarcoma* (Fig. 133-134)

This is the most important of the soft tissue tumours at this site. It occurs particularly in infants, children, and young adults.

In some cases cross-striations of the neoplastic cells are readily recognized on staining either with haematoxylin and eosin or with phosphotungstic acid haematoxylin. In others, less differentiated, there may be no demonstrable striations but characteristic rounded cells with eosinophilic cytoplasm may be found among the elongated spindle cells that form the bulk of the tumour.

2. *Others* (Fig. 135-138)

Of the other soft tissue tumours, lipoma, malignant fibrous histiocytoma, liposarcoma, fibrosarcoma, and leiomyosarcoma are the most common.

VIII. UNCLASSIFIED TUMOURS

These are primary benign or malignant tumours that cannot be placed in any other category.

IX. TUMOUR-LIKE LESIONS

A. Epidermal [epidermoid] cyst (Fig. 57): A cyst lined by keratinized stratified squamous epithelium without skin appendages. The cyst contains keratohyaline material.

If the cyst is adjacent to a scar or a focus of a recognized type of tissue, it should be classified as teratoma. If it occurs alone, it should be classified as an epidermal cyst.

B. Nonspecific orchitis

Tumour-like enlargement of the testis may result from acute or chronic nonspecific orchitis.

---

[1] Enzinger, F. M., Lattes, R. & Torloni, H. (1969) *Histological typing of soft tissue tumours*, Geneva, World Health Organization (*International Histological Classification of Tumours*, No. 3).

C. Nonspecific granulomatous orchitis (Fig. 139)

Granulomas are present within degenerating tubules and also between the tubules.

D. Specific orchitis (Fig. 140-141)

Tuberculous orchitis is usually an epididymo-orchitis. Syphilitic orchitis, however, may be confined to the body of the testis. Other infections such as brucellosis and rickettsial and viral infections, e.g. mumps, may be mistaken clinically for tumours.

E. Malakoplakia (Fig. 142-143)

In this condition large histiocytes containing Michaelis-Guttman bodies are the predominant constituents. In some cases special stains, e.g., PAS, von Kossa, or iron, may be required to demonstrate the inclusions.

F. Fibromatous periorchitis (Fig. 144): A diffuse or focal fibroblastic proliferation, often hyalinized and generally following inflammation or trauma, which may simulate neoplasm.

G. Sperm granuloma (Fig. 145-146): A granulomatous lesion, usually in the epididymis, resulting from the extravasation of spermatozoa that sometimes occurs in the cord following vasectomy. There are numerous phagocytes containing spermatozoa.

H. Lipogranuloma (Fig. 147): A reactive sclerosing lesion due to the injection of oily material. It may simulate liposarcoma.

I. Adrenal rests (Fig. 148): Encapsulated nodules of adrenal cortical cells situated on the surface of the spermatic cord, in the region of the rete testis, or in the testicular parenchyma. These cells reproduce the architecture of the adrenal cortex.

J. Others

Other lesions that may simulate tumours are gonadal splenic fusion (Fig. 149), supernumerary testis, intratesticular haemorrhage, nodules of Leydig cells in the spermatic cord, mesonephric rests, Müllerian rests, and cysts of various types (e.g., mesothelial cysts (Fig. 150)).

INDEX

Unless otherwise stated, the preparations shown in the photomicrographs reproduced on the following pages were stained with haematoxylin-eosin.

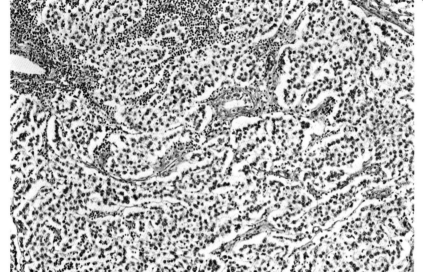

× 100

Fig. 1. Seminoma
  Lobular pattern. Lymphocytic infiltrate

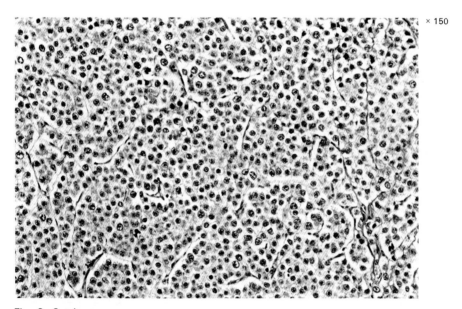

× 150

Fig. 2. Seminoma

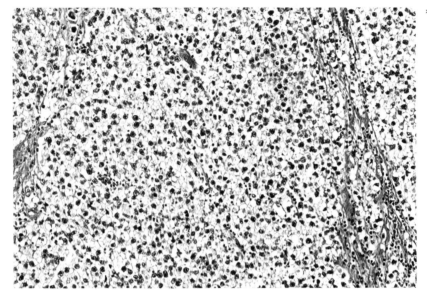

×130

Fig. 3. Seminoma
Clear cytoplasm. Well defined cell borders

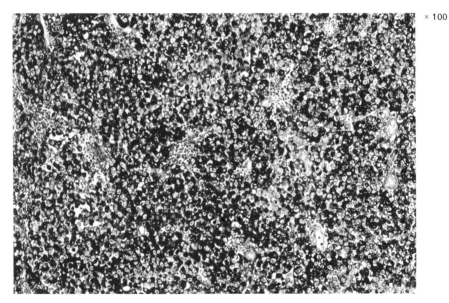

×100

Fig. 4. Seminoma
Abundant glycogen in cytoplasm. PAS

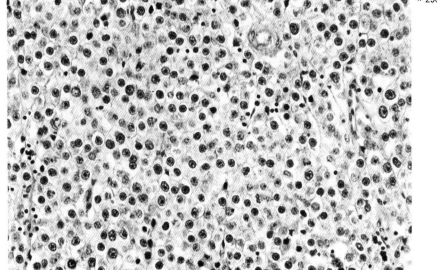

× 250

Fig. 5. Seminoma

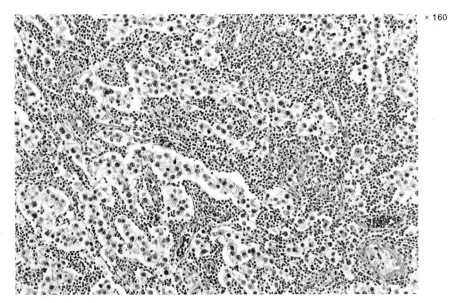

× 160

Fig. 6. Seminoma
Lymphocytic infiltrate

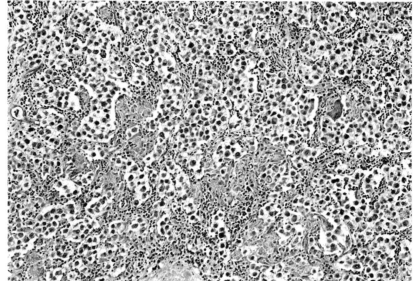

× 100

Fig. 7. Seminoma
Granulomatous reaction

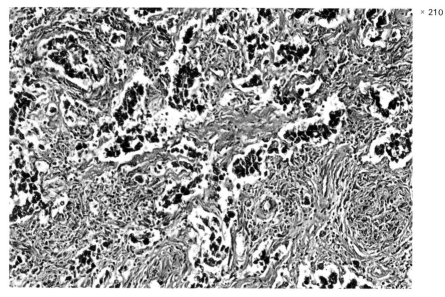

× 210

Fig. 8. Seminoma
Granulomatous reaction and extensive fibrosis

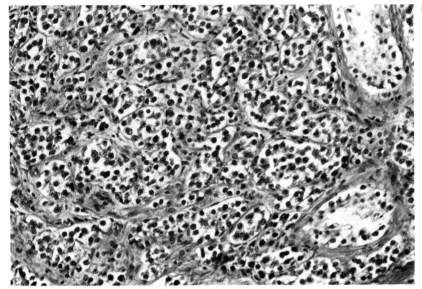

Fig. 9. Seminoma
Alveolar pattern

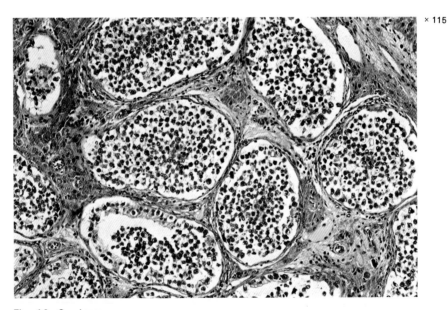

Fig. 10. Seminoma
Intratubular growth

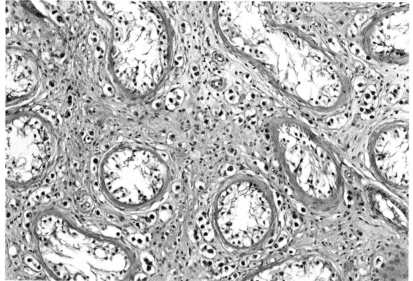

× 100

Fig. 11. Seminoma
Interstitial infiltration

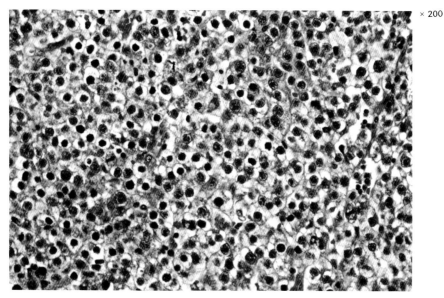

× 200

Fig. 12. Seminoma
Numerous mitoses

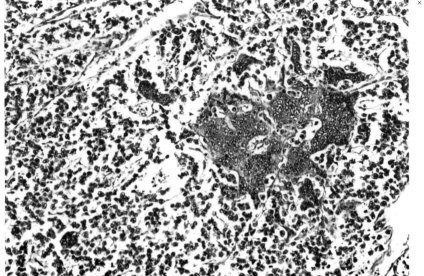

× 130

Fig. 13. Seminoma
Tumour giant cells

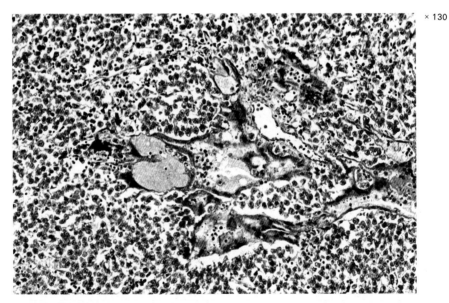

× 130

Fig. 14. Seminoma
Giant cells resembling syncytiotrophoblast

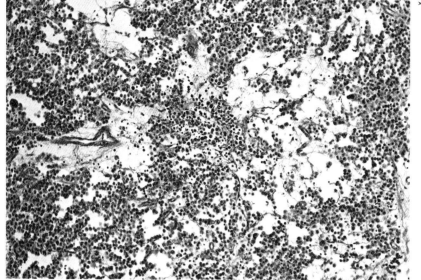

× 100

Fig. 15. Spermatocytic seminoma

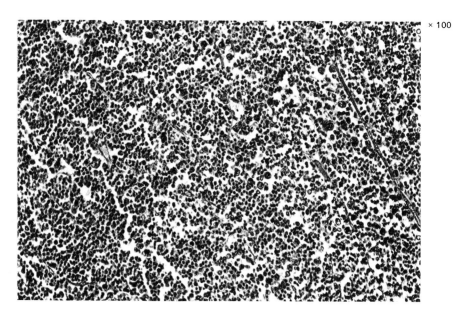

× 100

Fig. 16. Spermatocytic seminoma

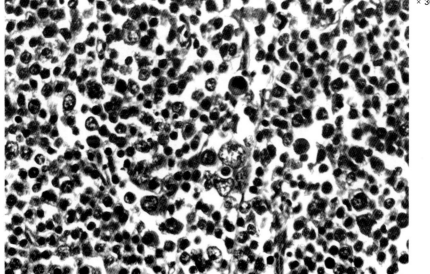

× 300

Fig. 17. Spermatocytic seminoma

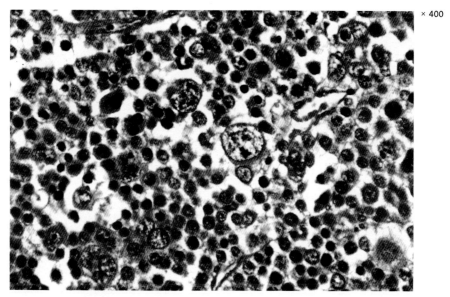

× 400

Fig. 18. Spermatocytic seminoma
Prominent variation in cell size

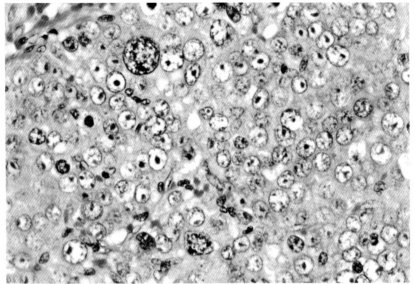

Fig. 19. Spermatocytic seminoma
Filamentous (spireme) chromatin pattern

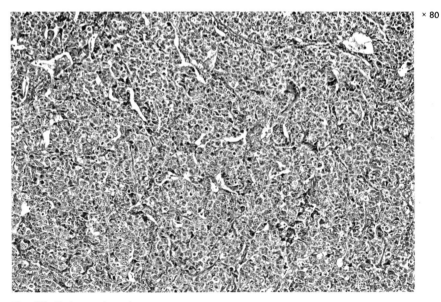

Fig. 20. Embryonal carcinoma
Solid pattern

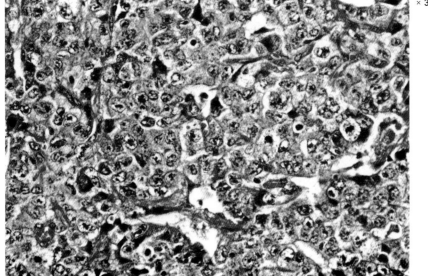

× 300

Fig. 21. Embryonal carcinoma
Solid pattern. Indistinct cell borders

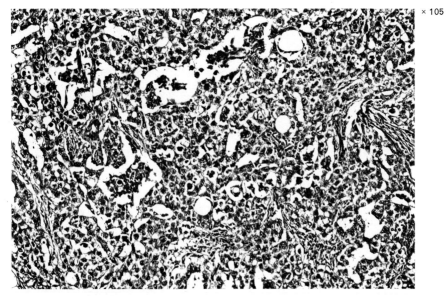

× 105

Fig. 22. Embryonal carcinoma
Solid and acinar patterns

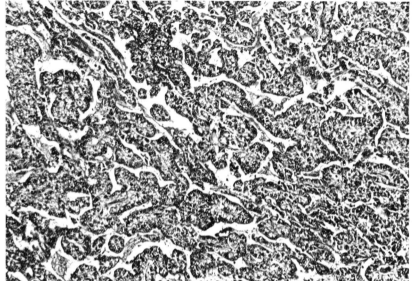

× 70

Fig. 23. Embryonal carcinoma
Papillary and tubular patterns

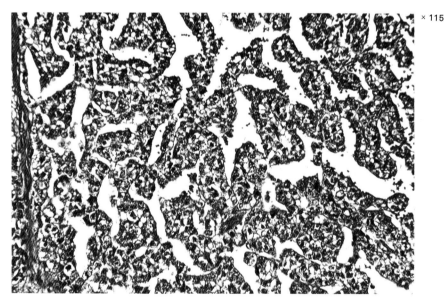

× 115

Fig. 24. Embryonal carcinoma
Papillary and tubular patterns

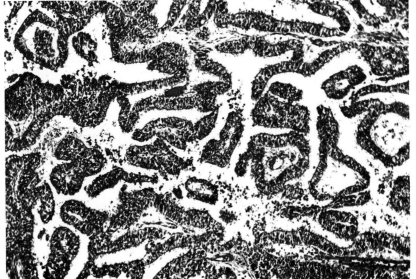

Fig. 25. Embryonal carcinoma
  Papillary and tubular patterns

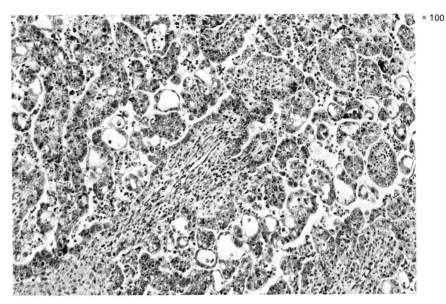

Fig. 26. Embryonal carcinoma
  Papillary and cyst-like structures

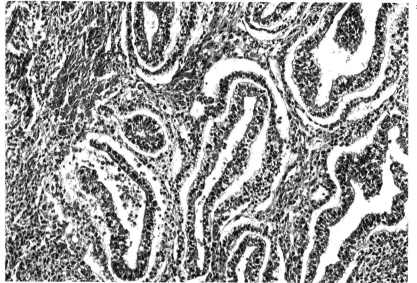

Fig. 27. Embryonal carcinoma
Double layered epithelium

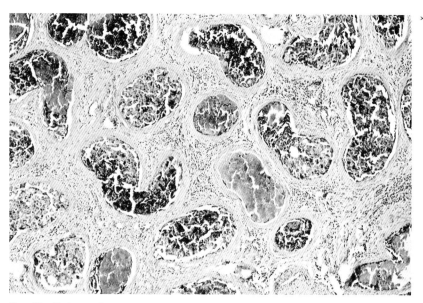

Fig. 28. Embryonal carcinoma
Intratubular growth with extensive necrosis

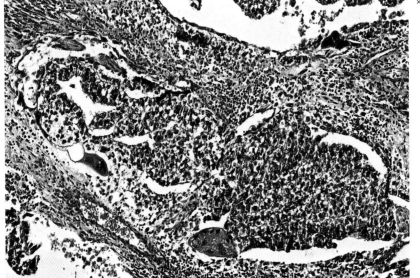

Fig. 29. Embryonal carcinoma
Giant cells resembling syncytiotrophoblast

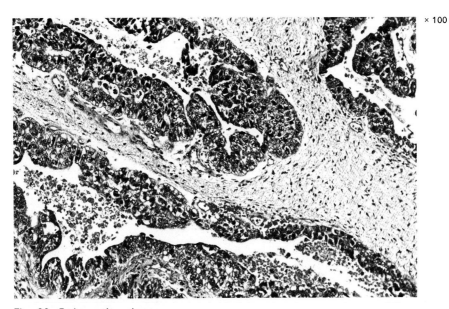

Fig. 30. Embryonal carcinoma
Primitive stroma

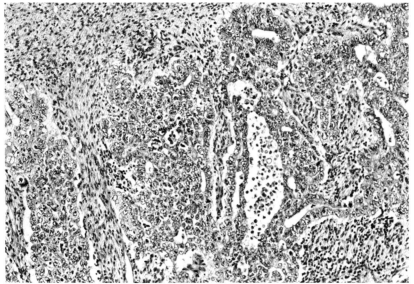

Fig. 31. Embryonal carcinoma
Primitive stroma

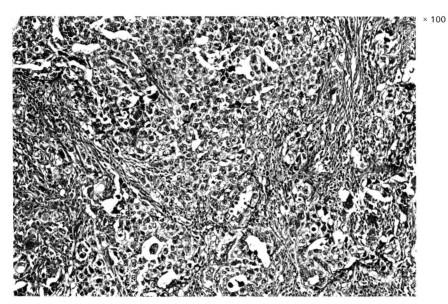

Fig. 32. Embryonal carcinoma
Granulomatous stroma

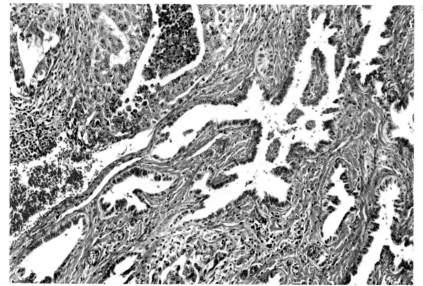

× 130

Fig. 33. Embryonal carcinoma
Extends to rete and simulates teratocarcinoma

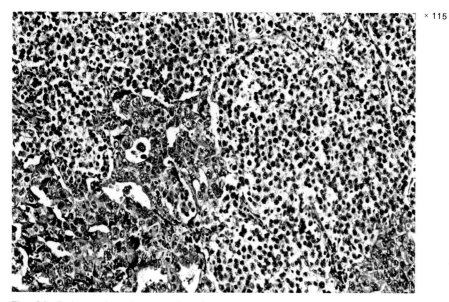

× 115

Fig. 34. Embryonal carcinoma and seminoma

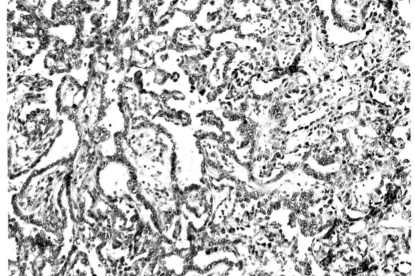

Fig. 35. Yolk sac tumour
Tubular and papillary structures

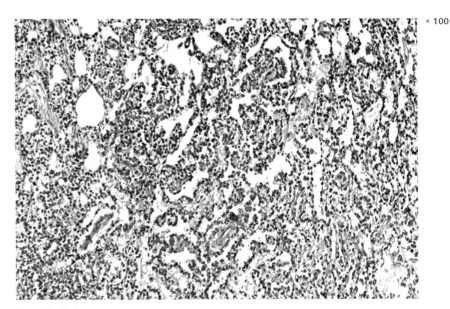

Fig. 36. Yolk sac tumour

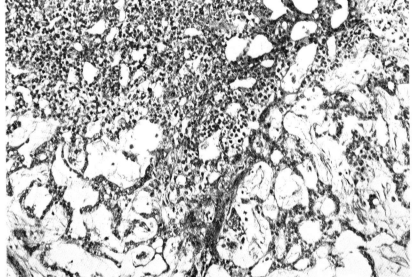

×110

Fig. 37. Yolk sac tumour
  Solid, tubular and reticular patterns. Adult patient

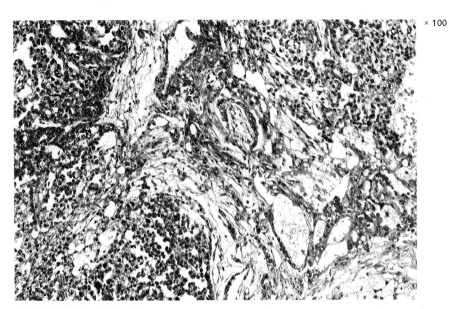

×100

Fig. 38. Yolk sac tumour

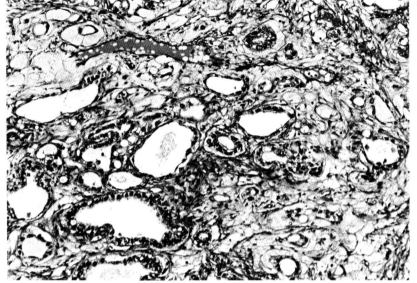

Fig. 39. Yolk sac tumour
Tubular structures and loose mesenchymal tissue

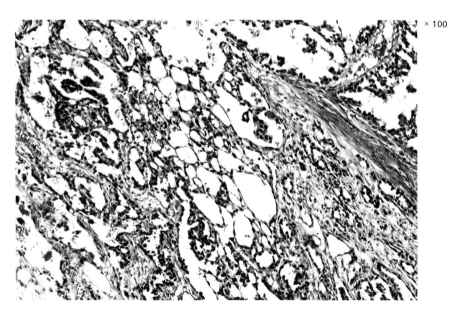

Fig. 40. Yolk sac tumour
Reticular pattern

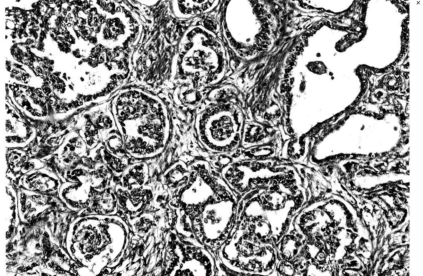

× 115

Fig. 41. Yolk sac tumour
Tubular pattern

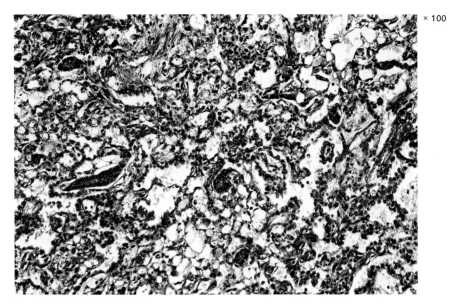

× 100

Fig. 42. Yolk sac tumour
Reticular and tubular patterns

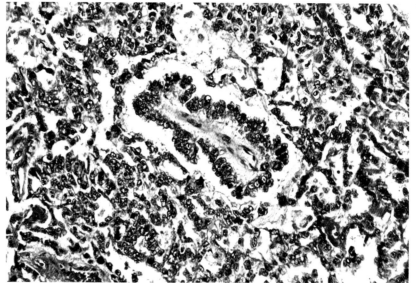

Fig. 43. Yolk sac tumour
Schiller-Duval body

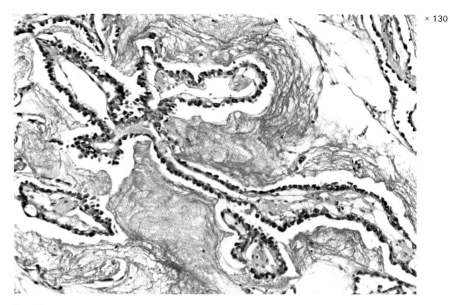

Fig. 44. Yolk sac tumour
Oedematous stroma

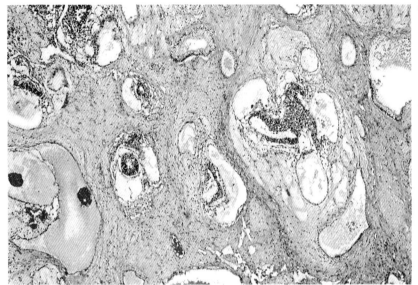

Fig. 45. Polyembryoma

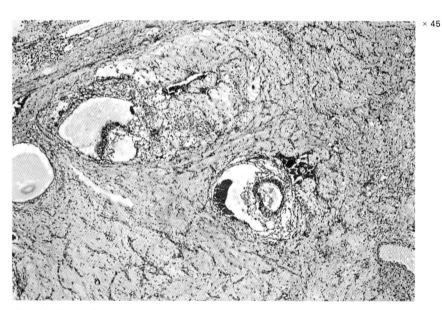

Fig. 46. Polyembryoma
Myxomatous stroma

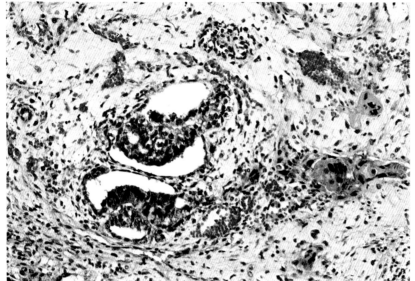

×150

Fig. 47. Polyembryoma
Embryoid bodies

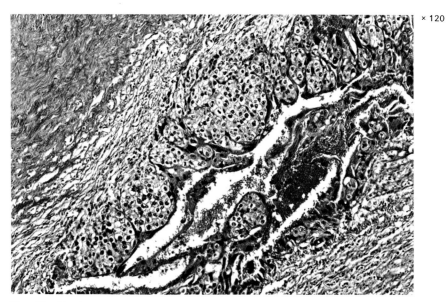

×120

Fig. 48. Choriocarcinoma

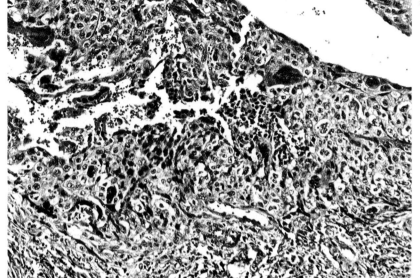

× 120

Fig. 49. Choriocarcinoma

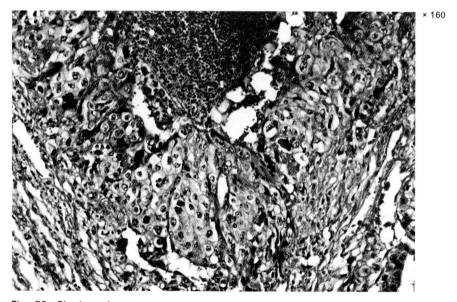

× 160

Fig. 50. Choriocarcinoma

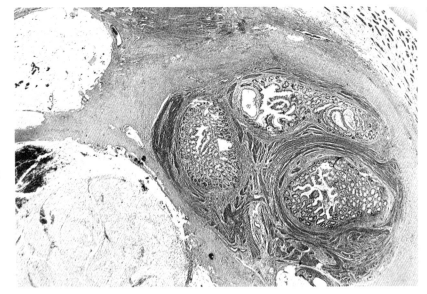

× 13

Fig. 51. Mature teratoma

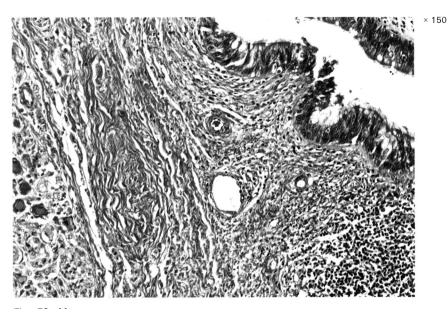

× 150

Fig. 52. Mature teratoma
Respiratory epithelium, ganglion cells and lymphoid tissue

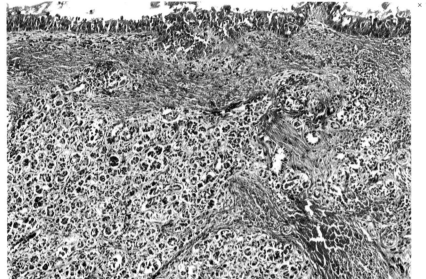

Fig. 53. Mature teratoma
Pancreatic tissue. Same case as Fig. 52

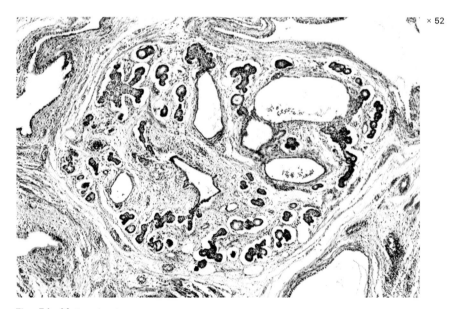

Fig. 54. Mature teratoma

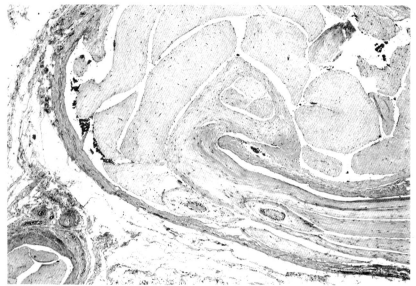

Fig. 55. Mature teratoma
Within spermatic vein

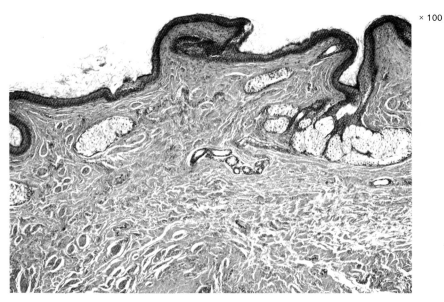

Fig. 56. Mature teratoma, dermoid cyst

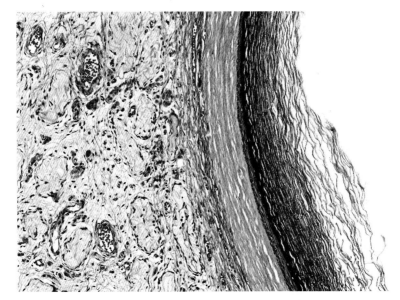

Fig. 57. Epidermal cyst

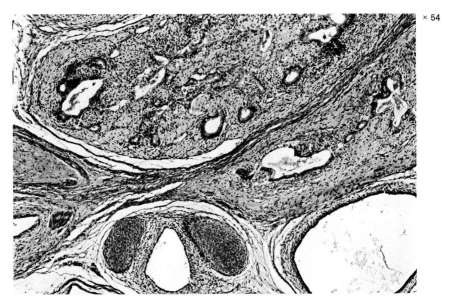

Fig. 58. Immature teratoma
Immature stroma and cartilage

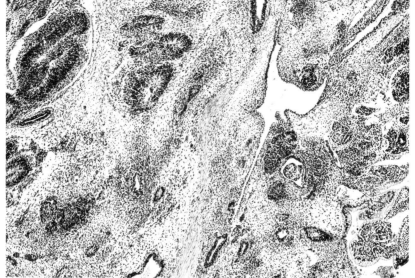

×48

Fig. 59. Immature teratoma

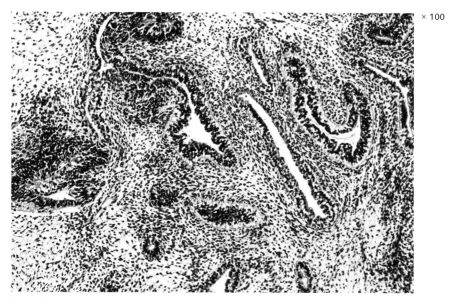

×100

Fig. 60. Immature teratoma

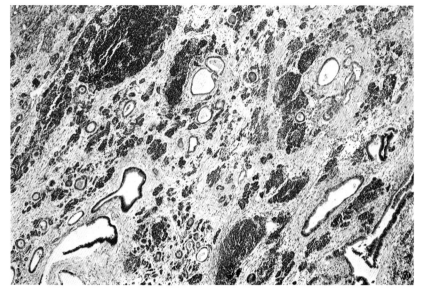

× 44

Fig. 61. Immature teratoma
Neuroblastoma-like tissue

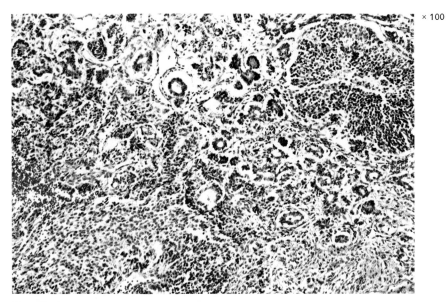

× 100

Fig. 62. Immature teratoma

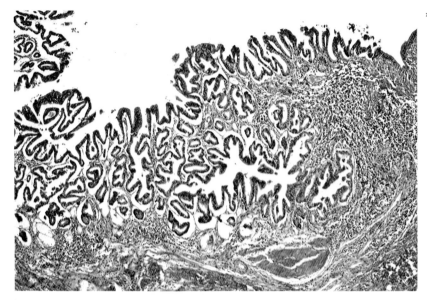

× 48

Fig. 63. Teratoma with adenocarcinoma

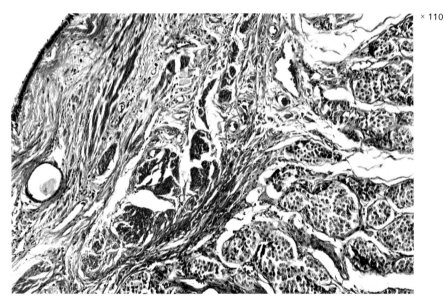

× 110

Fig. 64. Teratoma with carcinoid

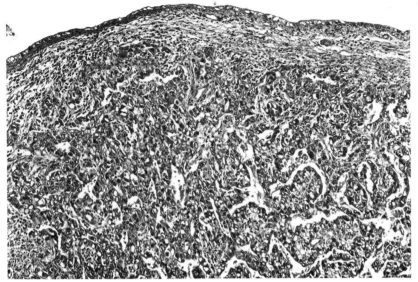

Fig. 65. Embryonal carcinoma and teratoma [teratocarcinoma]
Embryonal carcinoma beneath epithelial structure (teratoma)

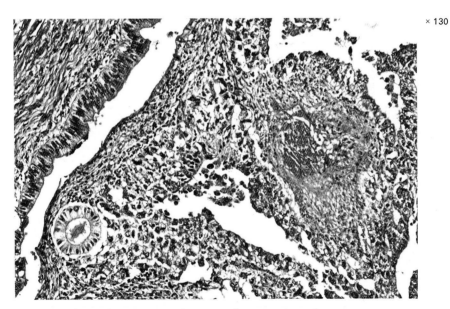

Fig. 66. Embryonal carcinoma and teratoma [teratocarcinoma]
Embryonal carcinoma at right, epithelium (teratoma) at left

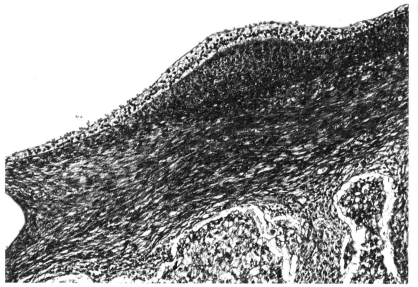

Fig. 67. Embryonal carcinoma and teratoma [teratocarcinoma]

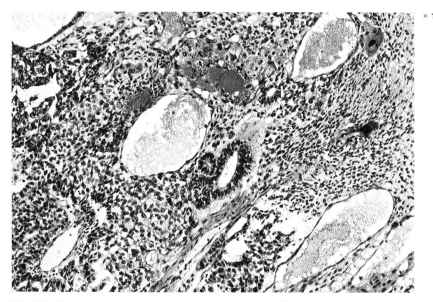

Fig. 68. Embryonal carcinoma and teratoma [teratocarcinoma]
Giant cells resembling syncytiotrophoblast

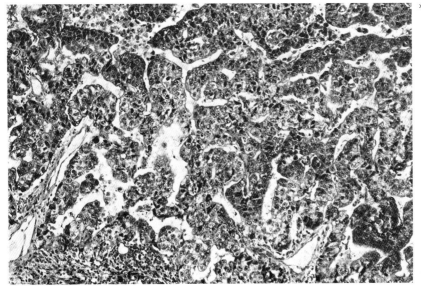

×115

Fig. 69. Embryonal carcinoma and teratoma [teratocarcinoma]
Same case as Fig. 68 with embryonal carcinoma component

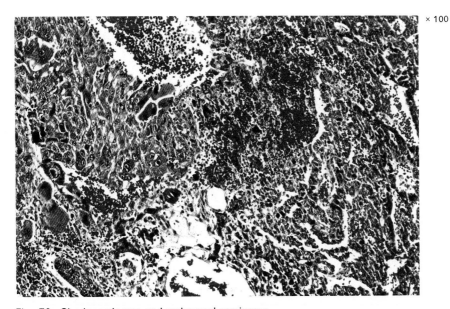

×100

Fig. 70. Choriocarcinoma and embryonal carcinoma

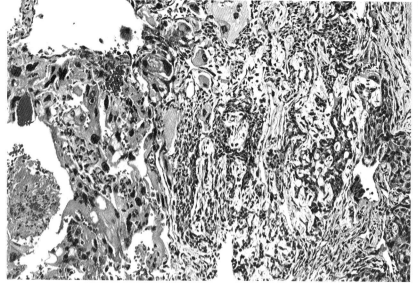

× 125

Fig. 71. Choriocarcinoma and teratoma

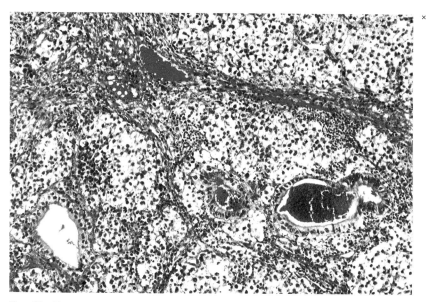

× 100

Fig. 72. Teratoma and seminoma

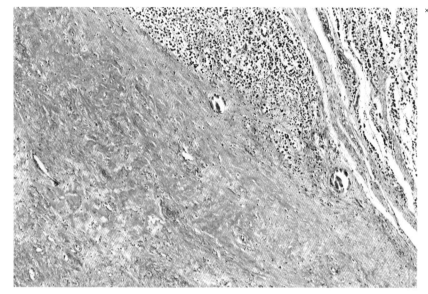

Fig. 73. Seminoma and scar

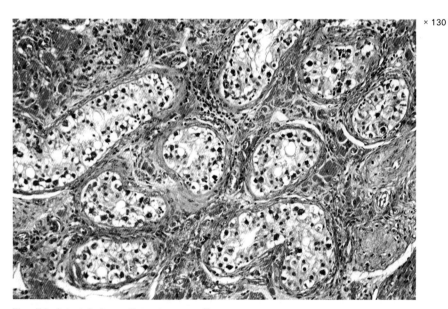

Fig. 74. Intratubular malignant germ cells

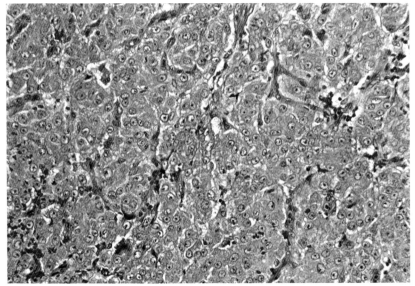

Fig. 75. Leydig cell tumour
Uniform cell population

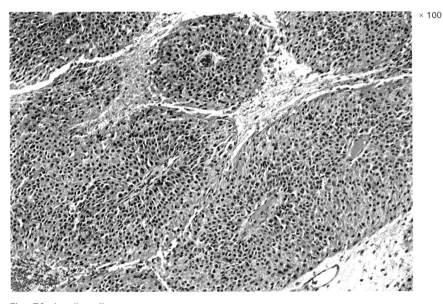

Fig. 76. Leydig cell tumour
Nodular growth pattern

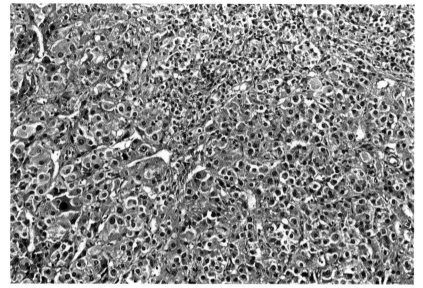

× 120

Fig. 77. Leydig cell tumour
Variation in cell size and shape

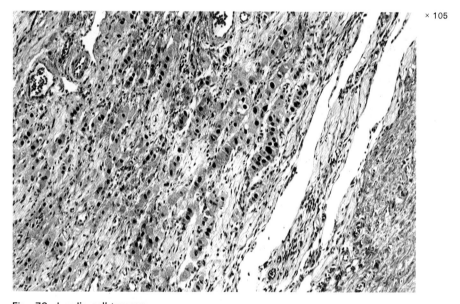

× 105

Fig. 78. Leydig cell tumour
Cells arranged in cords

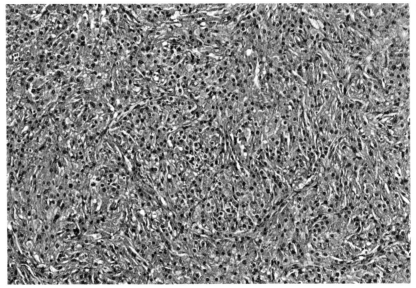

× 100

Fig. 79. Leydig cell tumour
Spindle shaped cells. Same case as Fig. 77

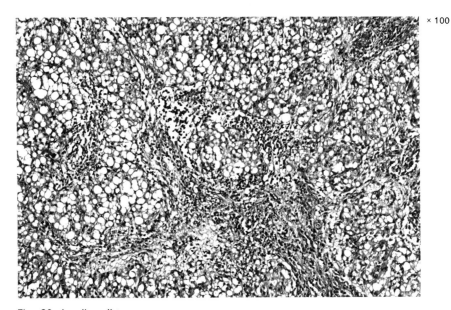

× 100

Fig. 80. Leydig cell tumour
Large cytoplasmic vacuoles

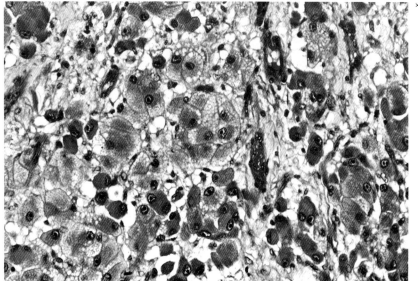

Fig. 81. Leydig cell tumour
Fine cytoplasmic vacuoles

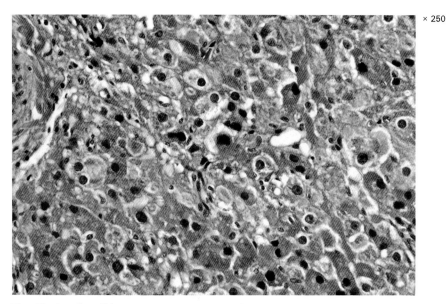

Fig. 82. Leydig cell tumour
Lipofuscin pigment in tumour cells

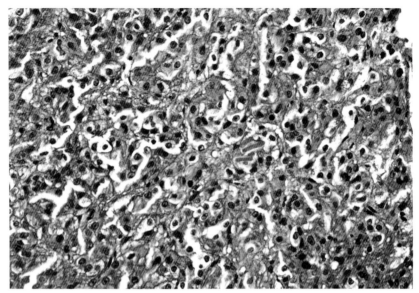

Fig. 83. Leydig cell tumour
Reinke's crystals

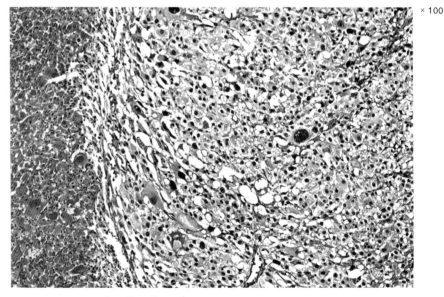

Fig. 84. Malignant Leydig cell tumour
Necrosis. Tumour metastasized

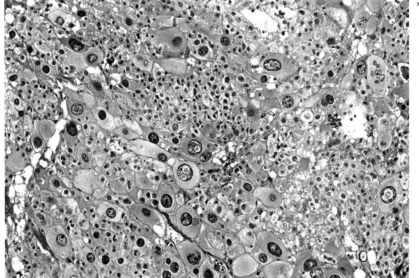

Fig. 85. Malignant Leydig cell tumour
Pleomorphism. Same tumour as Fig. 84

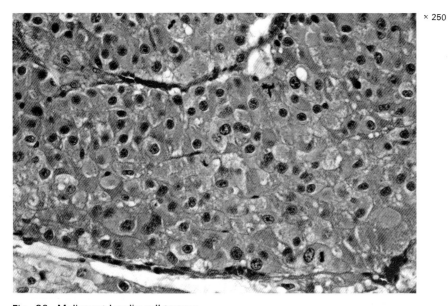

Fig. 86. Malignant Leydig cell tumour
Mitoses. Same tumour as Fig. 84

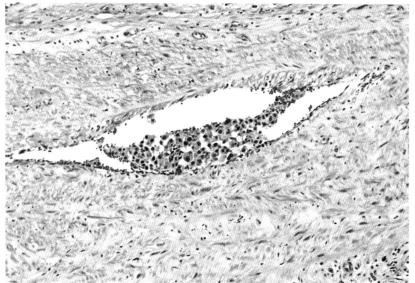

Fig. 87. Malignant Leydig cell tumour
Vascular invasion. Same tumour as Fig. 84

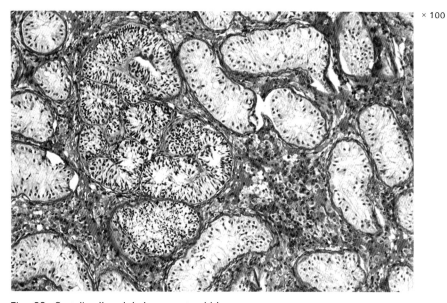

Fig. 88. Sertoli cell nodule in a cryptorchid

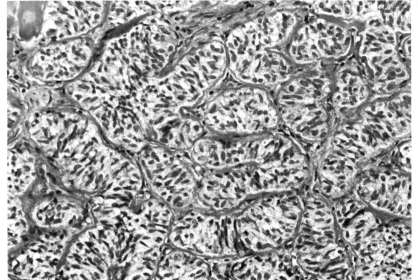

Fig. 89. Sertoli cell tumour

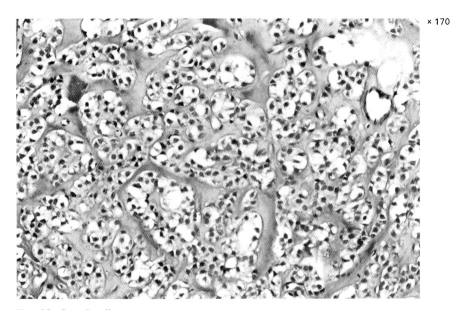

Fig. 90. Sertoli cell tumour
Hyalinized, thick basement membrane-like stroma

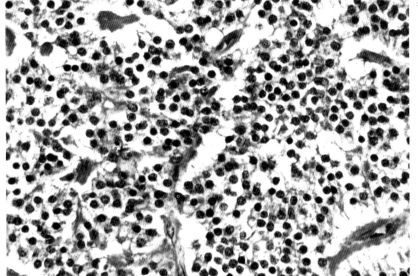

× 450

Fig. 91. Sertoli cell tumour

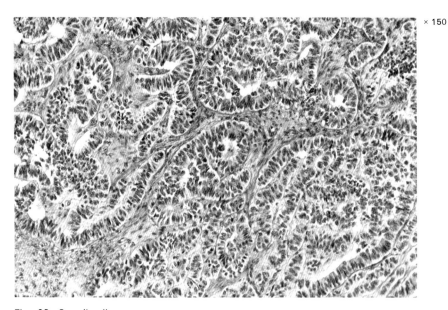

× 150

Fig. 92. Sertoli cell tumour
Ductal pattern

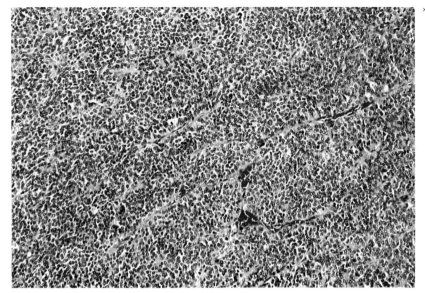

× 125

Fig. 93. Malignant Sertoli cell tumour
Tumour metastasized

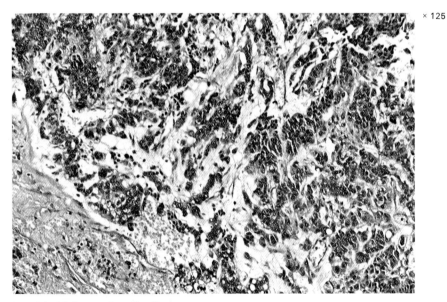

× 125

Fig. 94. Malignant Sertoli cell tumour
Same case as Fig. 93

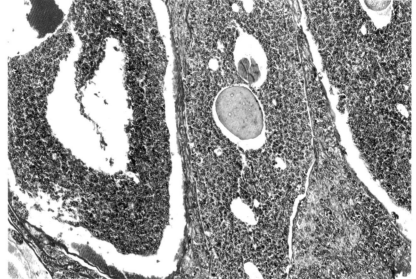

× 100

Fig. 95. Granulosa cell tumour

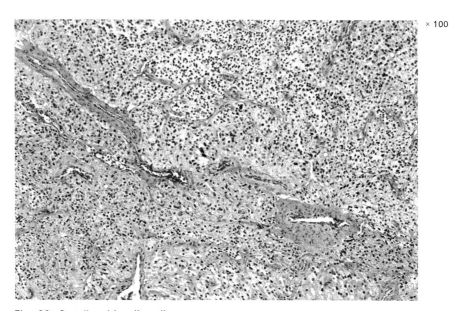

× 100

Fig. 96. Sertoli and Leydig cell tumour
Both cell types present

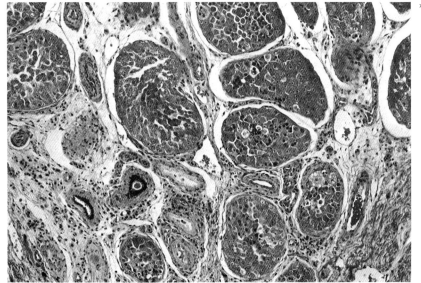

× 100

Fig. 97. Sertoli and Leydig cell tumour
Intratubular cells with eosinophilic cytoplasm resembling Leydig cells. Same case as Fig. 96.

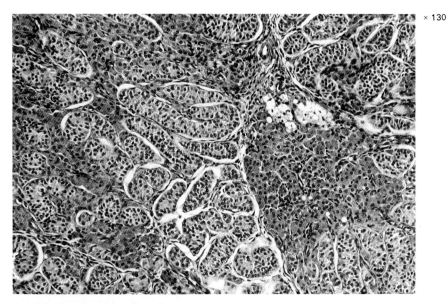

× 130

Fig. 98. Sertoli and Leydig cell tumour
Mixture of Sertoli and Leydig cells

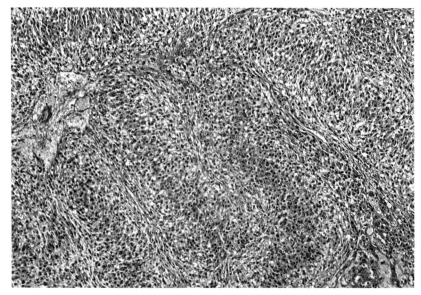

× 100

Fig. 99. Gonadal stromal tumour
Incompletely differentiated

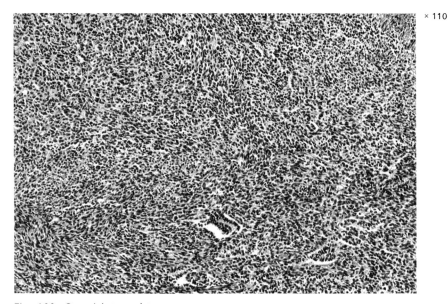

× 110

Fig. 100. Gonadal stromal tumour
Incompletely differentiated

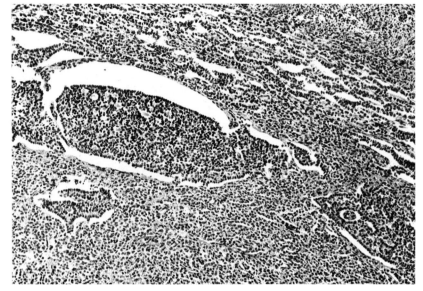

Fig. 101. Gonadal stromal tumour

Partial differentiation to granulosa cell elements. Same case as Fig. 100

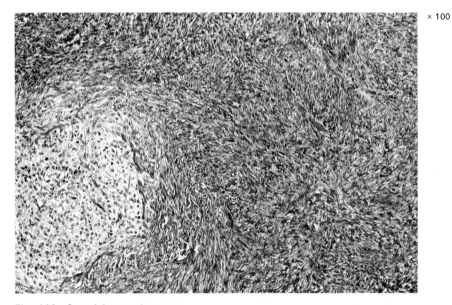

Fig. 102. Gonadal stromal tumour

Partial differentiation to theca and Sertoli cell elements

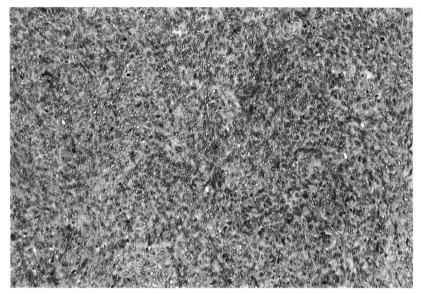

×170

Fig. 103. Gonadal stromal tumour
Incompletely differentiated

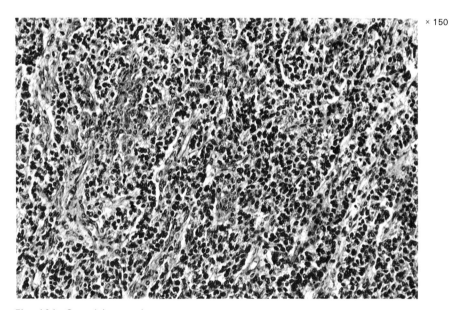

×150

Fig. 104. Gonadal stromal tumour
Incompletely differentiated. Tumour metastasized

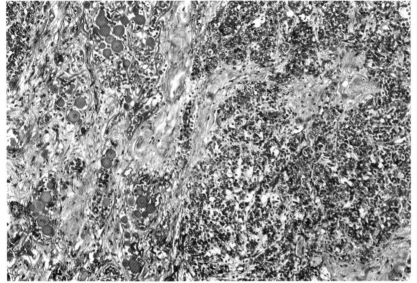

Fig. 105. Gonadal stromal tumour
Incompletely differentiated. Tumour metastasized

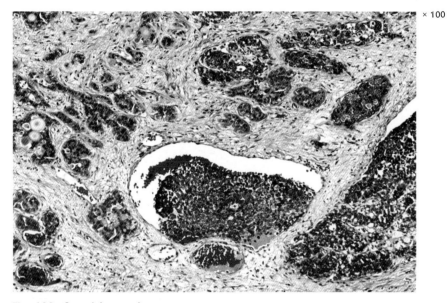

Fig. 106. Gonadal stromal tumour
Incompletely differentiated. Vascular invasion. Same tumour as Fig. 105

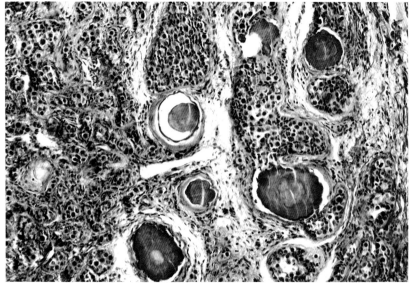

Fig. 107. Gonadoblastoma

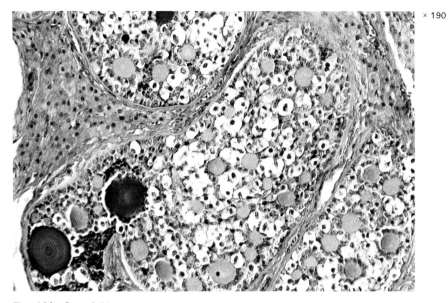

Fig. 108. Gonadoblastoma
Leydig, Sertoli and germ cells. Hyaline bodies and calcification

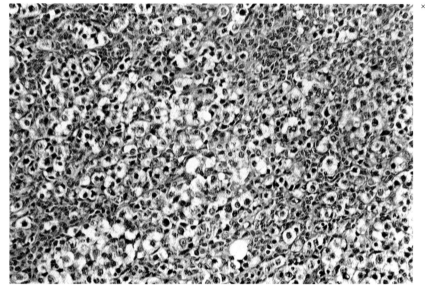

Fig. 109. Gonadoblastoma
So-called atypical gonadoblastoma

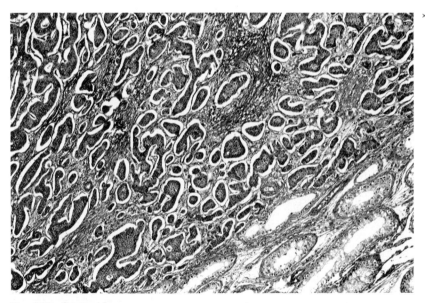

Fig. 110. Carcinoid
Primary in testis

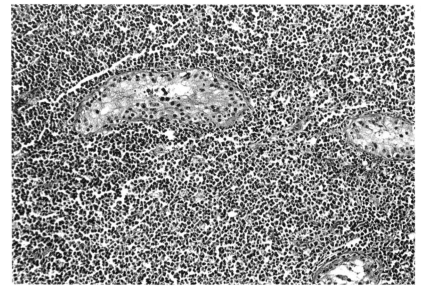

×100

Fig. 111. Malignant lymphoma

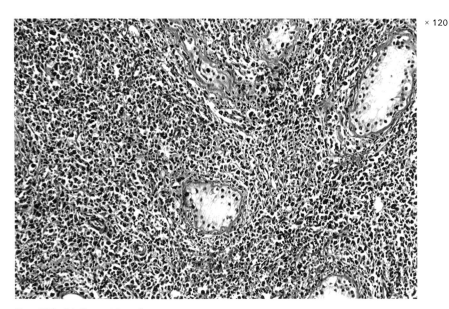

×120

Fig. 112. Malignant lymphoma

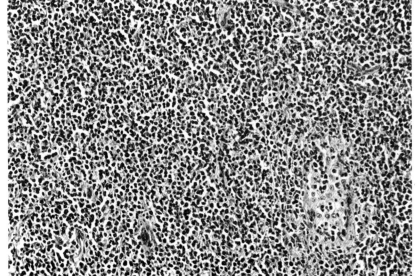

× 150

Fig. 113. Malignant lymphoma

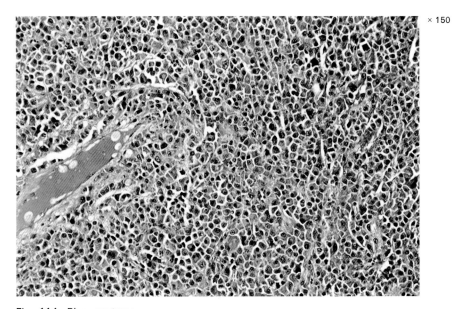

× 150

Fig. 114. Plasmacytoma

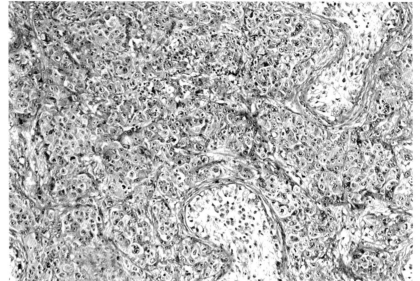

Fig. 115. Secondary tumour
Primary in lung

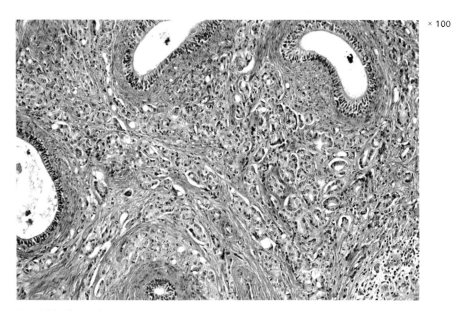

Fig. 116. Secondary tumour
Primary in prostate

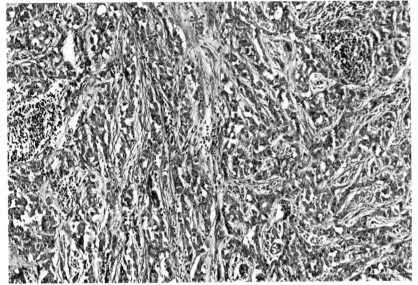

× 100

Fig. 117. Adenomatoid tumour

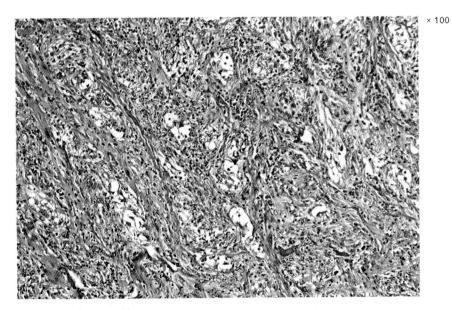

× 100

Fig. 118. Adenomatoid tumour

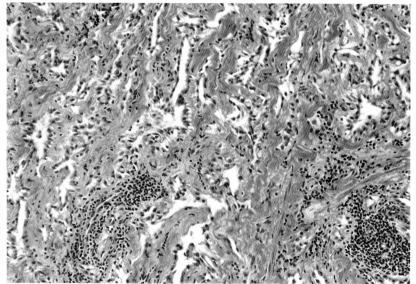

× 135

Fig. 119. Adenomatoid tumour

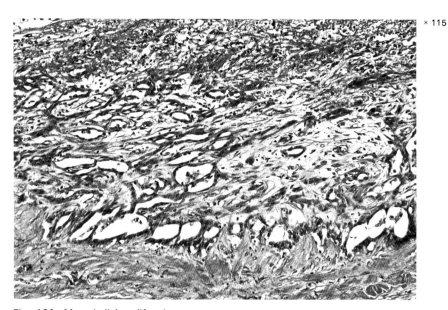

× 115

Fig. 120. Mesothelial proliferation

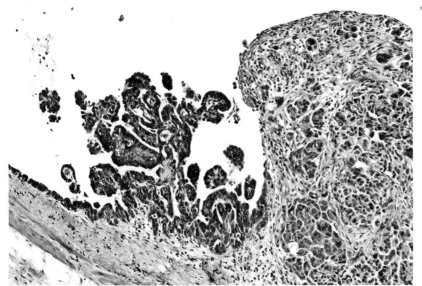

× 100

Fig. 121. Mesothelioma
Papillary and infiltrating. Malignant tumour in scrotal sac

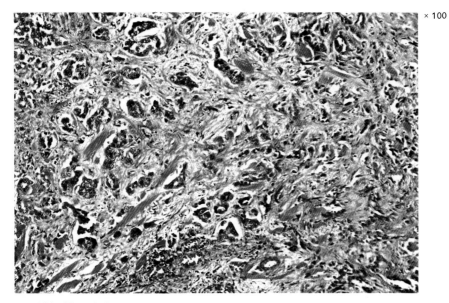

× 100

Fig. 122. Mesothelioma
Malignant

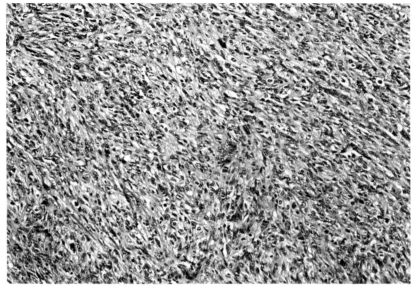

× 110

Fig. 123. Mesothelioma
Malignant. Spindle-cell pattern. Same tumour as Fig. 122

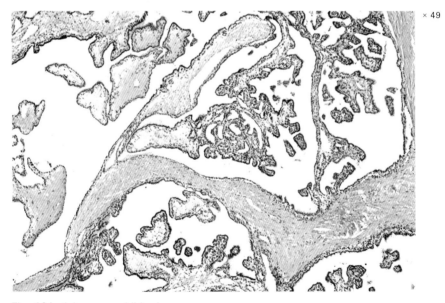

× 49

Fig. 124. Adenoma, epididymis
Papillary cystadenoma

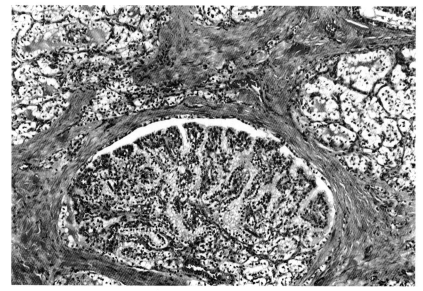

× 100

Fig. 125. Adenoma, epididymis
Glycogen-rich clear cells

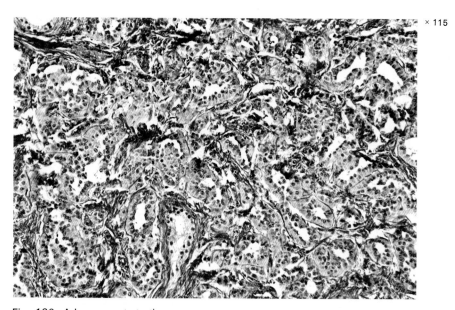

× 115

Fig. 126. Adenoma, rete testis

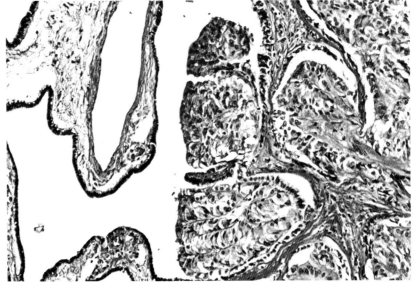

Fig. 127. Carcinoma, collecting ducts and rete testis
Resembles Sertoli cell tumour

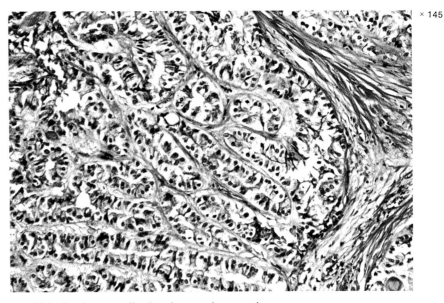

Fig. 128. Carcinoma, collecting ducts and rete testis
Same case as Fig. 127

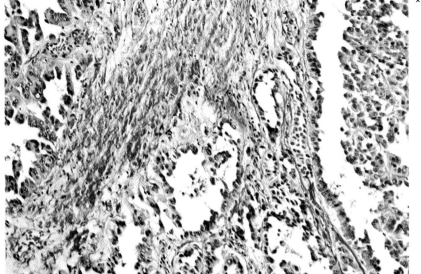

Fig. 129. Carcinoma, rete testis

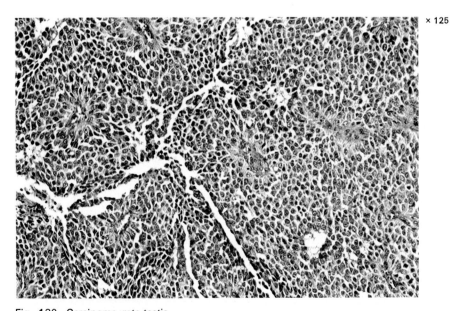

Fig. 130. Carcinoma, rete testis
Same case as Fig. 129

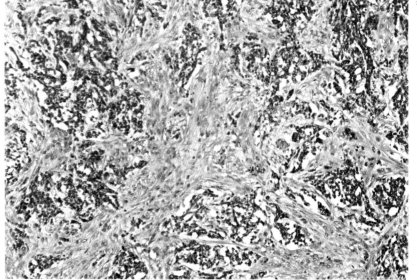

Fig. 131. Melanotic neuro-ectodermal tumour

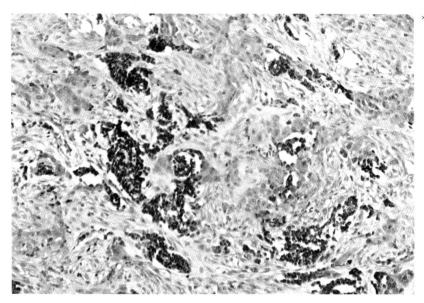

Fig. 132. Melanotic neuro-ectodermal tumour

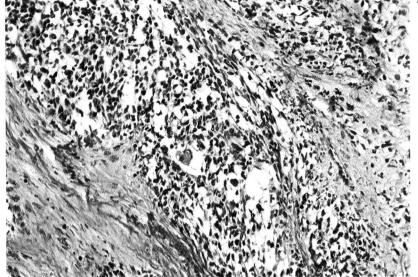

× 135

Fig. 133. Rhabdomyosarcoma, spermatic cord

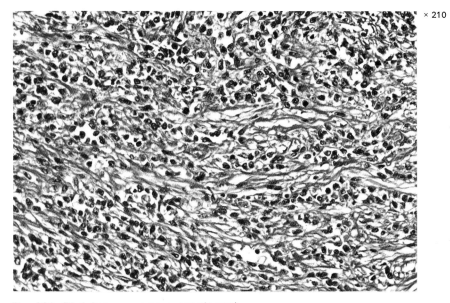

× 210

Fig. 134. Rhabdomyosarcoma, spermatic cord

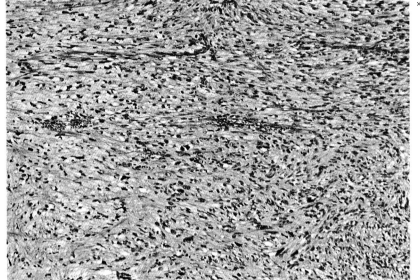

× 100

Fig. 135. Leiomyosarcoma, spermatic cord

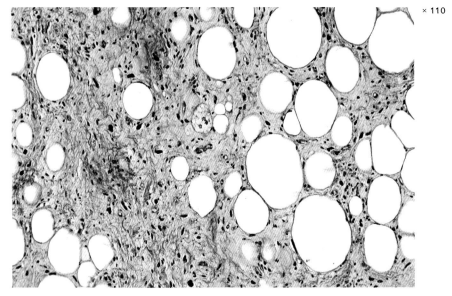

× 110

Fig. 136. Liposarcoma, spermatic cord

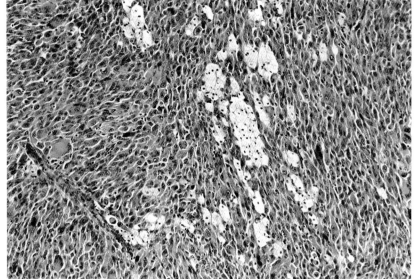

Fig. 137. Malignant fibrous histiocytoma

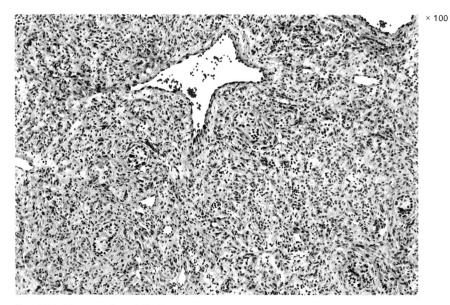

Fig. 138. Haemangioendothelioma
Several seminiferous tubules remain

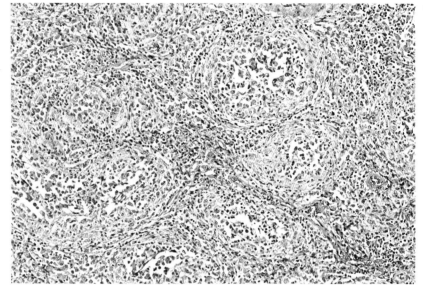

×100

Fig. 139. Granulomatous orchitis

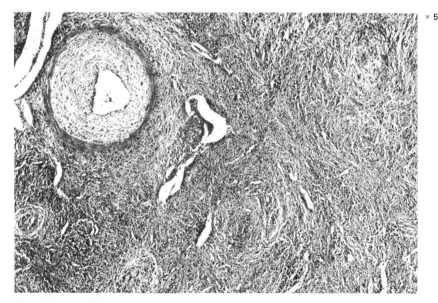

×50

Fig. 140. Syphilitic orchitis

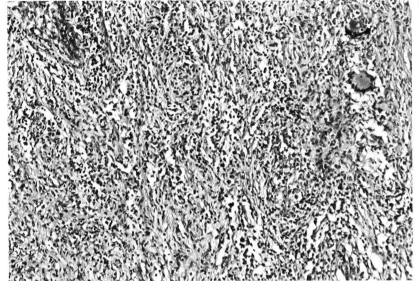

×110

Fig. 141. Syphilitic orchitis

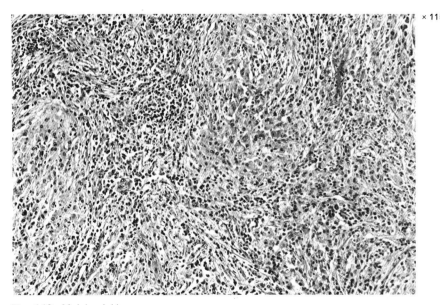

×115

Fig. 142. Malakoplakia
Granulomatous inflammation

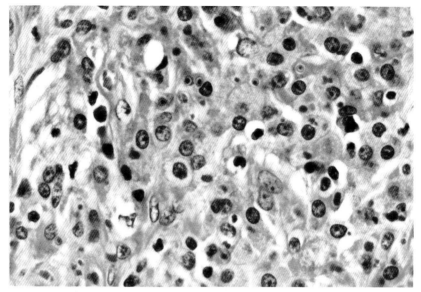

× 600

Fig. 143. Malakoplakia
Michaelis-Guttmann bodies

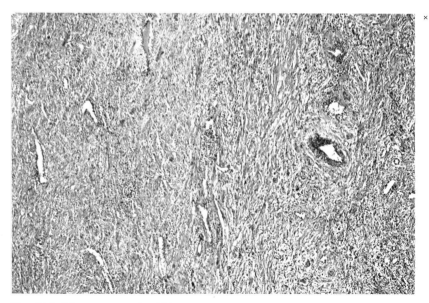

× 42

Fig. 144. Fibromatous periorchitis

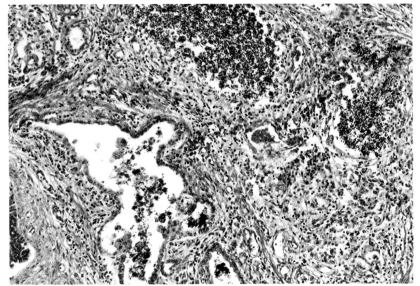

Fig. 145. Sperm granuloma

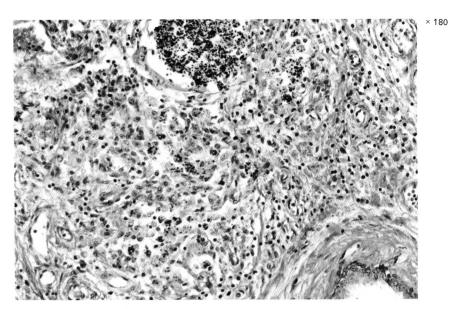

Fig. 146. Sperm granuloma
High magnification of Fig. 145

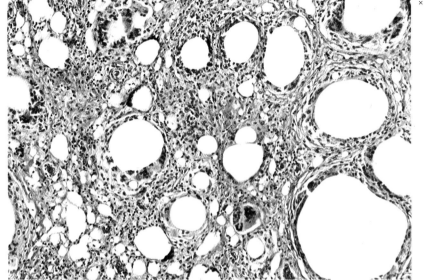

Fig. 147. Lipogranuloma, spermatic cord

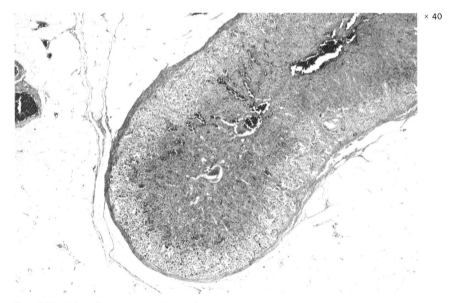

Fig. 148. Adrenal rest, spermatic cord

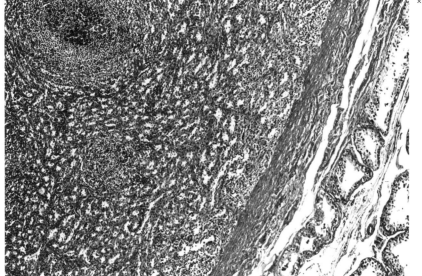

× 56

Fig. 149. Gonadal splenic fusion

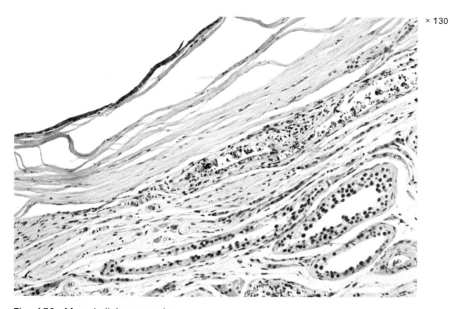

× 130

Fig. 150. Mesothelial cyst, tunica